The Longliving of Soviet Georgia

Professor G. Z. Pitskhelauri, M.D.

Director, Gerontology Center
Institute of Experimental and Clinical Therapy
Tbilisi, Georgia SSR

Translated and Edited by:
Gari Lesnoff-Caravaglia, Ph.D.
Sangamon State University
Springfield, Illinois USA

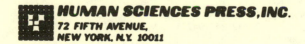

HUMAN SCIENCES PRESS,INC.
72 FIFTH AVENUE,
NEW YORK, N.Y. 10011

Copyright © 1982 by Human Sciences Press, Inc.
72 Fifth Avenue, New York, New York 10011

Printed in the United States of America
23456789 987654321

Library of Congress Cataloging in Publication Data

Pitskhelauri, G. Z.
    The longliving of Soviet Georgia.

    Translation of: Dolgozhiteli Gruzii.
    Bibliography: p. 142
    Includes index.
    1. Longevity—Georgian S. S. R.   I.   Title.
QP85.P5313   612'.68'094795   LC 81-4176
ISBN 0-89885-073-8   AACR2

Contents

List of Illustrations

Figures and Tables

Introduction

Gari Lesnoff-Caravaglia

Much interest has been generated in recent years by reports of persons living to advanced ages. One area of the world that has received a good portion of such attention is Soviet Georgia.

Although such world-wide attention has been intensified because of the increase in life expectancy throughout the industrialized world, interest in longevity and the extension of the life span has been of continuing interest to physicians and biologists in Soviet Georgia for several centuries.

In this edited English edition of *The Longliving of Soviet Georgia*, which originally appeared in Russian in the Soviet Union, Professor G. Z. Pitskhelauri traces this historical interest in longevity in Soviet Georgia and describes those areas of current Soviet research that focus upon aging and life extension. Professsor Pitskhelauri, a physician in his seventies, is Director of the Gerontology Center that conducted the research cited in this volume. Although the main Center for Gerontology of the Soviet Academy of Sciences is located in Kiev in the Ukraine, the Gerontology Center headed by Professor Pitskhelauri is in the heart of the region of the longliving.

Interest and research in life extension and longevity has been generally based upon technological advances and scientific expertise. In contrast, Soviet gerontologists increasingly stress the quality of life as the greatest asset to the increase in human life expectancy.

What is patently clear in the study of life-styles among the longliving (Pitskhelauri provides us with an entire daily schedule) is the element of continuity within the daily regimen, work habits, role expectations, and diet over extended periods of time. This is in sharp contrast to life-styles in much of the industrialized world which are based upon waves of shock from newness and sudden exposures. The harmonizing effect on both the psychological and physiological systems of such regulated existence, from which abrupt discontinuities are largely absent, minimizes shock to the organism and thus permits the enjoyment of long life.

The significance of harmony of both person and environment, which incorporates relationships with other persons, is the most significant finding in this present study of longevity. Living for long periods of time in one locality leads to the acclimitization of the human organism. Much like other animal species, the longliving blend with the landscape. The importance of the same geography, along with climatic conditions, is a new and fascinating concept.

The dilemma facing the modern age is one of fit between the increase in the life expectancy and the environment. Such lack of fit has resulted in the disastrous explosion of nursing homes, retirement villages, and geriatric hospitals. The deliberate separation of persons from the larger society has been legitimized on the basis of age, frailty, or illness. The normal condition of aging beyond societal expectations has led to ostracism.

Professor Pitskhelauri defines three categories of aging groups:

Mature	60–74 years old
Old	75–89 years old
Longliving	90 plus years old

Natural or physiological aging occurs at the age of 100 and above; premature or pathological aging occurs between the age of 60 and 70.

The concept of premature aging may be new to some industrialized nations, but this concept is closely linked to preventive medicine. This is a positive perspective because it denotes that, although aging is a natural process, it can be initiated before its time by improper health habits, insalubrious environments, and lack of significant social roles. Viewing aging before one's time from a scientific perspective as a result of external factors, is a new direction provided by Professor Pitskhelauri and Soviet gerontologists. This concept could be a stimulus for the development of a variety of preventive measures against premature aging throughout the world.

Professor Pitskhelauri presents a unique theory of aging. As a result of poor diet, poor environmental conditions, mental stress, or physical illness, the aging body becomes increasingly subject to disease. The organism may well have been able to withstand such stress in youth, but such original adaptability is gradually lost due to environmental factors that impinge on the internal order of the organism. Control of these external factors would lead to increased longevity, even without scientific intervention. This theory does not discount the possibility that with the aging of the organism new adaptive mechanisms may come into play that allow older persons to adapt anew to the multiple changes in the environment. Such external environmental factors, however, may be overwhelming in number and render ineffective the adaptive mechanisms. Physical changes and illnesses ordinarily associated with the aging process thus are often evidence of premature aging. Such age changes may also be viewed as disruptions in the normal adaptive mechanisms.

The human system is constantly influenced by a complex combination of environmental factors. If these factors are constant, the environment produces changes in the organism's physiological functions, generating a number of mechanisms of adaptation which enable the organism to exist in the given environment. The longliving people, in maintaining lives of continuity, have sufficient time for their adaptive mechanisms to function, thus they are able to live through illnesses which in other cultures are disabling.

The quality of everyday life exerts the greatest influence upon human physical and intellectual development, survival rate and the determination of life expectancy. Long life is also dependent on effective health care delivery systems and sophisticated medical technology. Unfortunately, we have fastened upon the latter to the virtual eclipse of the former. Although health care is an important aspect in any consideration of longevity, it remains only one aspect of the total configuration. Other areas of equal importance include economic well-being, meaningful social roles, moderation in diet, and an emphasis upon physical activity.

The current trend toward small families, divorce and separate living arrangements for each generation is in direct contrast to the life styles of the longliving. One of the most significant findings by Professor Pitskhelauri is that the presence of family members, of several generations, encourages continued social participation throughout the life span, as well as the opportunity to see oneself as part of a continuous human process. The pleasures and concerns of family life also serve to stimulate persons intellectually, spiritually and emotionally. Working long into advanced age is also regarded as a participation in family life, in the sense of contributing to its economic well-being.

The importance of childbearing in relation to longevity is a further new contribution to the literature by Professor Pitskhelauri. Women, he has found, who have large families, i.e., large numbers of children brought to term, are women who number among the long-living. Rather than serving as destructive elements in the physiological processes of women, pregnancy and childbearing are healthful aspects of development in the female organism.

Professor Pitskhelauri also makes reference to new areas of possible research. One such fascinating prospect lies in the analysis of zones of longevity. A determination not only in terms of the rural or urban distribution of longevous peoples, but in terms of particular altitudes above sea level. Such studies might well include the climate, solar radiation, ultraviolet radiation, geochemistry of the zone, as well as proximity of the sea.

What is increasingly clear is that it is not extraordinary age which occasions surprise, but rather the extraordinary lives led by persons in their nineties. Professor Pitskhelauri's descriptions point to the fact that these lives are meaningful and full of enjoyment until the moment of death. His study of the deaths of the longliving also indicates that the close of such lives often comes about with full knowledge of the dying person. They frequently conduct procedures of closure, such as final visits and the giving of final instructions before taking to bed and dying shortly thereafter.

Long life thus perceived is a complex combination of factors. It is this combination of climatic, geographic, ecological, and socioeconomic factors, together with heredity, that determine the ability to reach the biological limit of human life.

The benefits of a tradition that permits of a regulated and regular life style give us pause in the contemporary age, which is built upon change and the deliberate abandonment of tradition. We need to rethink the benefits of a traditional life style and the adoption of life styles foreign to our own that are often introduced through mass media. Such cultural imitation has seen its reflection in the appearance of the first retirement complexes, 12 stories high, on the skyline of Moscow.

1

Longevity

The Eternal Dream

Longevity and senescence are at the heart of the medical, biological, and social problems of contemporary society. The dream of prolonging human life, preserving youth, and postponing old age has irresistibly attracted humankind throughout history.

The search for "sources of eternal youth" and "immortality" has been the subject of numerous myths and legends, as well as the goal of fruitless searches by medieval alchemists. Seers and astrologers persisted in the attempt to find the route to longevity. Various remedies had been proposed by them, such as the "stone of immortality" and the "elixir of youth," along with numerous other talismans and amulets.

The Egyptians, in order to prolong life and preserve health, took purgatives and emetics for 3 days every month. Frequent sweating was recommended to eliminate harmful substances from the body through the skin.

The Greeks, on the other hand, resorted to more practical means. They believed that the intelligent use of natural factors was the most reliable means for preserving health and prolonging life. Hippocrates and the other Greek physicians recommended moderation and temperance in all things. They also urged the breathing of clean air, taking of cold baths, gymnastic exercises, and daily massage.

Although people of the past were limited in their abilities to improve life and to control premature senescence and diseases, or to conquer them, medical science throughout the world has made great strides in these directions. Many diseases that previously cost human lives have been eradicated. Effective means have been found for the treatment of illness, and drugs have been synthesized for the control of premature aging.

EARLY SCIENTIFIC STUDIES

A pioneer in the scientific study of the extension of the human life span was the Russian physician, I. B. Fisher (1685–1771). In his book, published in Latin in 1754, *On Old Age, Its Degrees and Diseases,* Fisher examined the physical conditions, the mental states, and the constitutional factors conducive to longevity. Through the use of autopsies, Fisher studied the age-specific changes in the organs of older persons. Among the important factors that lengthen life, I. B. Fisher cited the nervous system, as well as medical and hygienic procedures. The author emphasized the significance of emotional tranquility for the prolongation of life.

The well-known German scientist, Ch. Hufeland, in the foreword to his book, *The Art of Prolonging Human Life: Macrobiotics* (1796, p. 45) emphasized that the theory of "the art of prolonging human life" should constitute the contents of a special science, which he called macrobiotics. He wrote:

From this one can derive the appropriate hygienic and medical rules for prolonging human life which also constitute the subject of a particular science—macrobiotics, or the art of prolonging life. . . . The art of prolonging life should not be regarded as equivalent to ordinary medicine or medical dietetics; the latter have a different purpose, different remedies, as well as different parameters. The goal of medicine is health; the goal of macrobiotics is the extension of life. (p. 6)

In 1801 Parfeniy Yengalychev's four-volume treatise, *On Prolonging Human Life,* was published. The author of this voluminous work on the prolongation of life advised a strict adherence to dietetic laws; the timely treatment of disease; participation in physical exercise; abstinence from alcohol and nicotine; and the observance of personal hygiene.

The era of the complex clinicophysiological study of the phenomena of senescence and the processes of aging began with S. P. Botkin. The collection, analysis, and summarization of data on the almshouses in St. Petersburg (Leningrad today) was undertaken upon the initiative of S. P. Botkin. This survey was carried out and subsequently published by A. A. Kadyan (1890). This work, as well as individual studies by other authors conducted under the leadership and on the initiative of S. P. Botkin, represents a significant contribution to the study of longevity with respect to the understanding of the various aspects of the physiology and pathology of aging, along with practical information as to preventive measures that should be undertaken.

The great Russian scientist, I. I. Mechnikov, is credited with initiating the experimental study of senescence. He created a comprehensive theory of aging that was a unique variant on the theory of autointoxication.

I. I. Mechnikov published his studies on longevity in 39 experimental reports and monographs and thus laid the foundation for serious experimental research on the processes of aging and death. The results of many years of research by I. I. Mechnikov were published in his classical works: *Studies on the Nature of Man*, *Studies of Optimism*, *Prolonging Life*, and *A Forty Year Search for a Rational World View*. I. I. Mechnikov in pointing out practical methods for the control of premature aging, gave first priority to a balanced life-style as a requisite for longevity—orthobiosis.

A substantial contribution to the subject of longevity and aging was made by the great physiologist and scientist, I. R. Tarkhnishvili. His studies of longevity and extensive literature search appear in his magnum opus, *Longevity in Animals, Plants and Humans* (1891). He described the development of animals and plant organisms, the various human patterns of physiological functioning according to age, the processes of aging; and he provided recommendations for the prevention of senescence to ensure the prolongation of human life.

In 1901, I. I. Mechnikov introduced the term "gerontology," and in 1909, I. L. Nasher the term "geriatrics," to identify an independent medical specialty analogous to pediatrics. However, as early as the end of the 19th century (1891), I. R. Tarkhnishvili understood the urgent need for the establishment of a science dedicated to the prolongation of human life as an independent discipline. Tarkhnishvili saw the importance of developing a special division of medicine—gerontology—to study those factors that either shorten or promote the extension of life.

"Of course, hygiene," he wrote,

> which studies the prevention of disease, and practical medicine, which has as its goal the curing of disease, promote the preservation of life. At the same time, however, they lose sight of a large group of phenomena related to human longevity. The study of such phenomena should be mandatory in order to encourage the development of a special branch of science dedicated to the exploration of conditions which foster longevity. Unfortunately, nothing like this exists, and this, of course, is unfortunate for humankind (Tarkhnishvili, 1891, p. 10; for more details, see Pitskhelauri, 1968).

Much attention had been devoted by I. P. Pavlov to the study of particular features of the higher nervous activity exhibited in old age. He believed that

> the duration of human life should be no less than 100 years, and if many do not reach this age, this is only because they themselves, by intemperance, abuse of their own body, reduce this normal term to a much lower figure (Pavlov, 1949, p. 30).

In the first decades of the century, studies in the field of gerontology were greatly broadened due to the studies of I. P. Pavlov and his followers, among whom figured A. A. Bogomolets, A. S. Dogel, M. S. Milman, Z. G. Frenkel, A. V. Nagorny, N. D. Strazhesko, I. V. Davydovsky, N. N. Gorev, D. F. Chebotarev, V. N. Nikitin, and V. V. Alpatov.

Among Soviet hygienists who contributed to such studies were F. F. Erisman and Y. A. Osipov.

CURRENT RESEARCH

In the Soviet Union extensive gerontological research is being conducted, focusing on those aspects of the aging process that favorably or unfavorably influence life expectancy. Additional research is being conducted on new pharmacological agents that will benefit general body functioning and will prevent premature aging.

According to demographic projections, and the 1970 All-Union census of the USSR population, the numbers of older persons in both the mature and old categories will significantly increase in the near future. Such increases will bring about a number of serious socioeconomic and medical problems that will require immediate attention.

On the one hand, such needs will serve to intensify existing problems with respect to longevity and old age. On the other, they will encourage medicobiological, experimental, and clinical research.

The first USSR conference on the problem of the genesis of old age and the prevention of premature biological aging was held in December 1938, in Kiev. This conference, instigated by A. A. Bogomolets and organized by the Institute for Clinical Physiology of the USSR Academy of Sciences and the Institute of Experimental Biology and Pathology and Clinical Medicine of the Ukraine, had great significance for the development of gerontology and geriatrics in the USSR.

Extensive experimental and clinical material was presented at this conference, describing the physiological and pathological aging processes and the problems confronting medical science and public health in the field of gerontology ("Senescence," 1940).

At the 12th session of the USSR Academy of Medical Sciences, which was held in 1958, the basic trends in the development of longevity and senescence in the USSR were further delineated and discussed.

A planned development of gerontology and geriatrics in the USSR became possible with the creation of the Institute of Gerontology in Kiev in 1958, under the direction of the USSR Academy of Medical Sciences. Further growth and development was fostered by the attention of the All-Union Problem Commission upon the national significance of Gerontology and Geriatrics. The Kiev Institute for

Gerontology, now headed by academician D. F. Chebotarev, is presently an international base of the World Health Organization (WHO) for the training of gerontologists in the social and medico-biological problems of longevity and senescence.

The All-Union Scientific–Medical Society of Gerontologists and Geriatricians, organized in 1963, joining more than 20 scientific societies, is presently a member of the International Association of Gerontology. Geriatric centers for intervention and the prevention of premature aging and for increasing the life expectancy now operate in many cities.

In recent years, numerous scientific conferences and symposia have been held. Research institutes and various laboratories participate in the study of the problem of longevity and aging. Gerontological centers, institutes, laboratories, and a network of geriatric institutions have been created in many parts of the world as well. The International Association of Gerontology now includes 35 national organizations of gerontologists.

THEORIES OF AGING

Since the origin of the first scientific ideas on aging and human longevity, more than 200 theories have been developed that attempt to identify the causes of aging and the processes responsible for the age-specific changes in the organism. None of these hypotheses, however, can totally explain the complex mechanisms contributing to the aging process.

What does contemporary medical science have to say concerning aging and the causes of death?

Science distinguishes two types of senescence: natural senescence—that is, physiological aging—which occurs at ages in excess of 100 years; and premature senescence—pathological aging—which occurs earlier, between the ages of 60 and 70 years.

In the case of physiological aging, one can observe regular, progressive age-specific changes. Premature aging can be attributed to disease states as well as to a number of factors that are the result of unfavorable external and internal environments ultimately affecting the mechanisms that regulate the normal course of physiological aging.

According to I. P. Pavlov, the central nervous system, chiefly the cerebral cortex, plays the leading role in the aging process. His theory has led to investigations on the cellular, molecular, and submolecular levels.

The classic studies of Soviet biology dealt with the aging processes on a strictly biological basis, specifying the age-specific changes at all stages of ontogenesis and at varying stages of the life cycle. Subsequent investigations showed that the primary mechanisms of aging, which are characterized by a certain stability, are related to the genetic apparatus, that is, to the biosynthesis of protein.

During aging, the synthesis of ribonucleic acid (RNA) declines and significant changes occur in the genetic apparatus of the cell as the result of programmed shifts controlled by the so-called biological clock. The researchers Chebotarev, Frolkis, and Mankovski state that:

> The genetic apparatus of the cell contain complicated self-regulating systems for the biosynthesis of protein. This is why the analysis of the effect of the neurohumoral regulation on the processes of protein biosynthesis has acquired the greatest importance for the analysis of the role of age-specific changes in the regulatory systems on the state of the other tissues (1969, p. 9).

Since the strength and adaptive capabilities of the organism weaken with age, certain of its functions are extinguished. When elderly people suffer from certain diseases, their original ability to adapt may be lost. However, new important adaptive mechanisms come into play that allow older persons to newly adapt to the multiple changes in the environment.

The problem of scientists consists in studying these mechanisms that regulate the vital processes, discovering their origin, and applying them in aggressive and selective intervention procedures. Equally important is the study of the pathogenesis, the clinical picture, as well as the prevention and treatment of the diseases of the elderly. These diseases, it is clear, have their own specific features.

In the USSR, research emphasis has been placed on the complex study of the healthy organism at different periods of the life cycle, during both natural or physiological aging and premature or pathological aging (see distinction above). Along with the search for the biological principles responsible for human longevity, scientists are seeking to develop a pharmacology of aging. Significant research efforts are also devoted to studies of a sociohygienic character, and to the study of the life-styles of longliving persons. The role and significance of the sociohygienic research has grown, especially during the past 2 decades.

In this connection, new branches of gerontology have been developed: social gerontology, which studies the social aspects of aging; and gerohygiene, which studies a number of hygienic disciplines as they relate to the three aging categories: the mature, the old, and the longliving.

There is no doubt that societal expectations play as significant a role with regard to the extension of the human life span as do biological states. It is well to bear in mind, however, that a further increase in human life expectancy is based not only on a gradual change in hereditary makeup—an extremely slow process—but upon social conditions as well. It is precisely the socioeconomic status— the quality of everyday life, living conditions, nutrition, and financial security—that exerts the greatest influence upon human physical and intellectual development, survival rate, and the determination of life expectancy.

Z. G. Frenkel wrote:

> The problem of long life, prolonging life in human society, is based upon a complicated set of social relationships within the total social structure. From what originally appears as a purely biological problem inevitably results in a socio-historical, and subsequent socio-hygienic question (1949, p. 81).

It is important to bear in mind that human life expectancy, like mortality, depends to a great extent upon effective health-care delivery systems and the level of sophistication of medical technology.

SOCIAL AND ECOLOGICAL RESEARCH

Ecological factors such as work habits, diet, nutrition, adequate housing, and general living conditions, as well as the climatic and geographic setting, cannot be ignored. The growing interest in social and ecological research in gerontology has been documented by increasing research efforts, publications, and scientific meetings dealing with these topics on both national and international levels.

An example of such growing concern is that at the eighth meeting of the International Association of Gerontology in Washington, D.C. (1969), approximately 95 reports on social gerontology were presented. At the ninth meeting in Kiev (1972), the total number of such reports exceeded 200. This testifies to the heightened interest of scientists in social gerontology and its significance in dealing with senescence and human longevity.

In Georgia, USSR, the first studies on social gerontology were initiated in 1955. In 1956, the monograph, *The Oldest People of Tbilisi*, was published. This broad-gauge study examined the lifestyles of persons who lived to advanced age in the city of Tbilisi (Shapiro, Pitskhelauri, & Gagua, 1956).

In the Georgian SSR, a republic of high longevity, studies on the problems of longevity and senescence have been greatly expanded in the past decade. According to the data of the All-Union Problem Commission on gerontology and geriatrics, the Georgian SSR is second in the world in terms of numbers of studies conducted in this field, following the Ukranian SSR, which is first.

Because of the major role of social and environmental factors in health and life expectancy, a division of gerontology was instituted in the N. I. Makhviladze Research Institute for Industrial Hygiene and Occupational Diseases in Tbilisi in 1951. This office undertook a study of a broad range of social problems related to longevity and senescence. Included in these studies were the effect of environmental factors upon older persons of all categories in both home and work situations.

The division of Gerontology subsequently developed into the Georgian Gerontology Center, which has conducted a large-scale study of persons aged 80 years and older throughout the republic.

Under the leadership of the Gerontology Center, other studies have been instigated in other centers organized in the autonomous republics of Abkhazia and Adzharia, as well as the south Ossetian autonomous province.

In 1962, the Center, which had been renamed the Social-Hygienic Gerontological Laboratory, was transferred to the I. F. Zhordania Research Institute for Human Generative Function of the Ministry of Health of the Georgian SSR. With the development of this laboratory, the All-Union Problem Commission on gerontology and geriatrics decided to establish a transcaucasian section of this commission in Tbilisi. This section was to coordinate the scientific research being conducted in the transcaucasian republics.

In 1959, the Tbilisi Research Medical Society of Gerontologists and Geriatrists was founded, and in 1965, the Republic Society. Societies of the same name were established in Sukhumi and Batumi.

Approximately 15,000 persons aged 80 years and older have been examined in the Social-Hygienic Laboratory for Gerontology. Following the model developed by the Kiev Gerontology Institute, the study includes the distribution of longevous persons by climatic and geographic areas. A map of population density of older persons was compiled and published in the *Atlas of Georgia* by the Academy of Sciences of the Georgian SSR (1965), together with materials on the census of 1959.

Residential, cultural, and hygienic conditions; family status and marital status; childbearing capability of women, and sexual potency of men; level of work activity, state of health, diet, and other aspects of the life-styles of the longliving persons were studied. Equally important studies were conducted on the socio-demographic characteristics of the older age groups of the population and the causes of invalidism and mortality of persons of the older age groups within urban settings. Additional areas of study included: the hygienic evaluation of living conditions, the state of health and occupation of those under the care of homes for the disabled and elderly of Georgia, the cardiovascular morbidity throughout the areas where the longliving were to be found, morbidity with temporary loss of working capacity of advanced-age workers of the tobacco factories, the motor activity and heart pathology of the persons reaching 80 years and older, the diet, and the effect of longevity on the generative and reproductive function of women. The complex clinicolaboratory study of the functional status of the cardiovascular system of persons between the ages of 90 and 114 years and living in rural regions of the republic has also attracted a certain amount of scientific interest.

Methods have been developed in the laboratory for the accurate determination of the ages of longliving persons. Proposals for the creation of a network of geriatric institutions have been generated, as well as procedures for classifying the work and recreational opportunities in homes for the disabled and elderly. Geriatric studies are also being conducted in the Research Institutes for Experimental and Clinical Therapy, the Research Institute for Experimental Morphology of the Georgian Academy of Sciences through its gerontological division, the Department of Hospital Surgery of the Tbilisi State Medical Institute, and in the Sukhumi Republic Hospital.

2

Medieval Medical Practitioners in Georgia

The Prevention and Treatment of the Diseases of Old Age

In the works of medieval physicians of Georgia, problems with regard to the prevention of premature senescence and the principles of treatment of disorders found in advanced age are given significant attention (for more details, see Pitskhelauri & Dzhorbenadze, 1969). Along with such practical work, these physicians wrote scientific treatises in which they provided a definition of medicine, its theory and practice. The causes of disease are described, as well as the basic principles of prophylaxis, diagnostics, and treatment of disease. These early writings laid the foundation for medical thought in Georgia and delineated the scope and technique of the medical arts.

In the treatise *Ustsoro Karabadini* by Kananeli, physician and researcher of the 11th century, one finds descriptions of the biological changes in the aging organism, information on the pattern of diseases in the elderly, and recommendations for proper nutrition in old age, as well as information on life expectancy. Kananeli divides human life into four age periods: childhood, youth, maturity, and senescence—which, in his opinion, begins after the age of 52.

During the senescent period, according to Kananeli, of the four body fluids, phlegm or mucus ("balgami") predominates. It is the quality of phlegm—coldness and wetness—which the author views as the nature of old persons. These same fluid properties condition the occurrence of all other biological changes in old age. The author describes in detail the characteristic physical and psychological features of senescence: graying of the hair, loss of teeth, absence of appetite and consumption of a small amount of food, general weakness, reduction in visual and auditory acuity, senile dementia, and reduction in sexual potency (Kananeli, 1940, pp. 39–40).

In contrast to such early developmental classifications, the age periods accepted by contemporary gerontologists transpose the period of senescence from 52 years in Georgia of the 11th century to 75 years in the present day.

Kananeli was also familiar with the concept of "premature aging." He discusses this concept from the perspective of the theory of the four bodily fluids that was accepted by medieval medicine.

Kananeli goes on to say that the older organism undergoes changes in the direction of an increase in "coldness and wetness." Following Hippocrates, he states that aging is the result of the loss of "congenital heat," and that the elderly are not only cold but also wet. As the "fire is removed from them and water flows in, dryness is destroyed and moisture is restored" (Hippocrates, p. 456). The author's understanding of aging as a process of hydration of the organism clearly establishes his writing in the preavicennian era. He was obviously not familiar with the principles of physiology and pathology of Ibn-Sina, who expressed in his "Canon" the idea of the dryness of the senescent organism. Subsequent studies in this field also indicate that "man of advanced age displays a tendency toward intracellular dehydration, whereas the extracellular space is in a state of slight hyperhydration" (Binet & Bourlier, 1960, p. 448).

In delineating the lung diseases to which older persons are frequently subject, Kananeli describes the gravity and duration of such conditions. He also notes the ineffectiveness of therapy resulting from the reduced quantity of "inborn heat" in the elderly organism, which is insufficient to control the disease.

In a chapter on the formation of stones in the kidneys and urinary tract, the author of *Ustsoro Karabadini* details the clinical picture and therapy of nephrolithiasis. His findings that stones are formed more frequently in the kidneys in old persons, but in the bladder in children, corresponds to the data of contemporary urology.

At the same time, the author attempts to establish the etiology of nephrolithiasis: "The stone arises from food consisting of buttermilk; fresh and unsalted, as well as aged cheese; crushed groates, dry bread; and the drinking of cloudy water and thick wine." (p. 339) Contemporary urology, as is known, ascribes a certain significance to diet and hard, salt-rich drinking water as factors promoting the development of nephrolithiasis.

An example of the contemporary nature of some of the statements in this treatise is the author's treatment of insomnia among the elderly. He proposes a number of hypnotic agents to prevent this condition. "Sleep is necessary and beneficial for the elderly; it is the source of health and strength," writes Kananeli (1940, p. 418). This observation on the beneficial effect of sleep on the elderly organism has received corroboration in contemporary studies.

Because of his understanding of the particular nature of the aging organism, Kananeli separated the elderly into a distinct group and differentially prescribed medication. For example, in the chapter on the benefit and possible harm of bathing procedures, he provides guidelines for bathing, encouraging its moderate use by aged persons, alluding to the harmful nature of frequent and long baths. With regard to diet, the author recommends river fish and fresh mutton, and encourages abstinence from pickled and salted meat (Kananeli, 1940, p. 190).

Among the medical achievements of Georgia during the feudal period was the work *Tsigni Saakimoi* (Kopili, 1936). Its 13th-century author was Khodzha Kopili. The author ascribed great diagnostic importance to the study of the pulse of young and old people. "The pulse of the elderly is sparce (slow) and uneven, . . . " writes Khodzha Kopili (1936, p. 38). As is known, bradycardia and limitation of the pulse parameters are, from the standpoint of contemporary cardiology, inevitable clinicophysiological features of senescence.

The ability of the Georgian doctors of the Middle Ages to make a macroscopic analysis of the urine merits attention; they were well aware of its changes with age. "The urine of the young is thick, while that of the elderly is colorless and fluid," writes Khodzha Kopili. (p. 40) His observations coincide with the contemporary view that the external appearance of the urine in old age reflects the processes of physiological aging in the kidneys.

Of the diseases of the genitourinary system to which elderly and senile persons are subject, the author of *Tsigni Saakimoi* describes disturbances in micturition, distinguishing between incontinence and urinary retention. Khodzha Kopili was well acquainted with the clinical picture of cystitis and considered involuntary micturition a manifestation of this disease in the elderly. He believed the cause for urinary retention to be the formation of tumors in the neck of the urinary bladder. This early observation agrees with current data indicating that up to 80% of men aged 80 years and older suffer from hypertrophy of the prostate gland.

The author's statement regarding the gravity of the prognosis and the hopelessness of the treatment of prostate hypertrophy, especially among the very old, also sounds quite contemporary. Therapeutic measures recommended by him for the treatment of urinary disorders include: the seeds of cucumbers and pumpkins; almond milk; plantain extract; fresh fennel and celery juice and other urologic agents; limitation of fluid intake; heat in the form of heating pads; and catheterization with a hollow reed.

The book contains no direct reference to the reduction in the total blood volume in the aging organism, but as the following quotation indicates, this change in the blood system, which is characteristic of the elderly, was known to the author. "When man has completed 60 years, bloodletting is unsuited for him, since the blood is reduced and emaciation will occur" (Kopili, 1936, p. 18).

The Armenian physician-scientist of the 12th century, Mikhtar Geratsi, was of the same opinion. He did not recommend the bleeding of weakened patients, particularly the elderly (Geratsi, 1968). The work of the 15th-century author Dr. Zaza Panaskerteli-Tsitsishvili, entitled *Samkurnalo Tsigni* (1950, 1959), also contains information of gerontological importance. Panaskerteli describes the incidence of kidney stone disease in persons of advanced age, drawing attention to such symptoms as pain in the lumbar region, hematuria, and the presence of a precipitate (sand) in the urine. According to Panaskerteli, old people are also subject to a skin disease in the form of a small-blister, highly prurient pox. This suggests chronic pemphigus vulgaris, which is frequently observed between the ages of 60 to 80 years.

Among the numerous prescriptions listed in *Samkurnalo Tsigni* is a formula for a complex medication the author recommends for persons of middle and old age. This is an amber decoction ("ambris gvarishni") made of 18 varieties of medicinal herbs: balsam oil; clove; the skin, seeds, and fruit of a number of plants; and honey. Some of the ingredients include spices or condiments, such as clove, cardamom, cinnamon, and pepper. As is known, the changes in the alimentary canal in old age assume the character of atrophic processes, which are accompanied by a reduction in gastric secretion and gastric juice acidity. The incorporation of these condiments in the remedies for the elderly, which improve digestion and intensify the secretion of the glands of the alimentary canal, is fully justified.

This corroborates current data on the diet of the longliving persons of Georgia, in which condiments and hot spices, which greatly improve the appetite and taste of foods, figure prominently. By and large, the amber decoction apparently exerts a tonicizing and rejuvenating effect on the aging organism.

In Zaza Panaskerteli's work there appears the following noteworthy statement: "People accustomed to heavy physical labor, the lifting of weights, are stronger than many untrained youths, even in old age" (1959, p. 93). The theory that work and systematic physical exercises strengthen the health and working capacity, increasing the body's ability to combat premature aging, has not lost its significance even at the present time.

The questions of longevity and senescence stimulated the interest of Ioane Bagrationi, an outstanding scholar-encyclopedist of the 18th century. M. Shengeliya discovered the voluminous manuscript, *Collected Medical Works of I. Bagrationi*, written in Georgian in the Leningrad Institute for Oriental Studies. On pages 469–474 of the collection appears a formula for an "elixir for long life." A compilation of books published in Russia in the 18th century by S.M. Grombakh, included a volume by an unknown author of the same title (Grombakh, 1953, p. 278). Further searching led to the discovery in a public library in Leningrad of the book listed by S. M. Grombakh, published in Russian by the St. Petersburg Provincial Government Printing Office and containing the original recipe for the "elixir of long life and its properties."

A comparison of the original Russian and Georgian texts of the formula showed that the Georgian version is a literal translation of the Russian. The translation was effected by I. Bagrationi in 1805, as confirmed at the end of the Georgian version of the formula and by the signature of I. Bagrationi himself.

The recipe for the elixir for long life contains a list of drugs used as ingredients, the method of their preparation, a list of diseases cured by the elixir, and the instructions for its use. The recipe includes drugs that increase digestive activity, stimulate the appetite, choleritic agents, laxatives, and so on. Judging by the ingredients, the elixir could exert a beneficial effect on the aging organism.

The unknown author of the formula writes that "the elixir enlivens the vital spirit, sharpens the senses . . . preserves the health and gives long life! . . . It may be called the restoration or the resurrection of humanity. . . ." The formula, it is reported, was found in the papers of the Swedish doctor Irnest Pernest, who died at the age of 104 from an injury sustained by falling from a horse. The ancestors of the doctor were also distinguished by remarkable longevity. The formula was passed on from generation to generation for many centuries.

A study and analysis of the major medical writings of the medieval period indicates that a rather high level of gerontological and geriatric knowledge had been achieved. Medical practitioners were aware of age differences, the need to categorize older persons into several groups such as mature, old, and longliving, as well as the prevention and treatment of premature aging.

The medieval Georgian medical practitioners also clarified issues

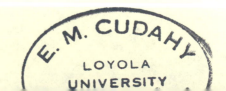

of gerontological dietology with recommendations concerning the acceptability or prohibition of one or another group of food products for older persons. The practical advice on personal hygiene, working conditions, sleep and waking, and physical exercises for the elderly also merit attention. Some of these recommendations hold true even in the present day.

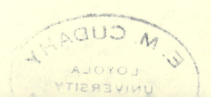

3

Soviet Georgia

A Republic of
Longliving People

Georgia is situated between the mountain chains of the Major and Minor Caucasus in an area of about 70,000 square kilometers. According to the data of the All-Union Census of 1970, more than 4,600,000 people live in Georgia. The republic includes the Abkhazian ASSR, the Adzharian ASSR, and the South Ossetian autonomous province.

Georgia is rich in sunshine and fertile lands, water bodies and healing mineral springs, forests and mountain pastures. In the fields, plantations, and gardens of Georgia ripen grapes, tea, citrus fruits, tobacco, sweet bay, tung, and many other varieties of fruit.

In Georgia are also located many health resorts and vacation recreation centers for workers. The health resorts of Tskhaltubo, Borzhomi, Gagra, Abastumani, and Pitsunda are widely known. Georgia presents a countryside full of contrasts. Within a relatively small area can be found a variety of climatic zones and landscapes from humid maritime subtropics on the coast to eternal snows and glaciers in the highlands. Such a surprising wealth and variety of natural surroundings is due, above all, to the geographic position, the complex terrain, and the altitude.

In the half-century of history of Soviet Georgia, many advances have been made in disease prevention and in the improvement of the health of the people. Such changes are due to improved economic and social conditions, as well as medical progress. Current health-care procedures include: service without charge, general accessibility of trained medical assistance, and widespread disease prevention.

Throughout Georgia are located 586 large hospitals, 1,449 polyclinics and outpatient clinics, 120 dispensaries, and 70 first-aid stations. In addition, there are 1,500 pharmaceutical establishments, 90 sanitary-epidemiological stations, and 22 research institutes dedicated to specific research areas. Medical care is provided by about 18,000 doctors, 3,000 pharmacists, more than 60,000 junior and intermediate medical personnel. For every 10,000 persons there are 36.3 doctors and 85.9 intermediate medical workers—a ratio unequaled in many parts of the world.

Recent health developments include an 1,100-bed clinic hospital in Tbilisi with the projection of specialized hospitals of 500 beds and more to be erected in Tbilisi, Sukhumi, and Kutaisi. Several large regional hospitals and other medical establishments are in the planning stage. More than 180 doctors and 700 medical science candidates are employed in the research institutes, in the 80 departments of the Tbilisi State Medical Institute and the Tbilisi Institute for Postgraduate Medicine. Leading Georgian physicians are active members and corresponding members of the USSR Academy of Medical Sciences and the Academy of Sciences of the Georgian SSR.

The health resorts of Georgia such as Gagra, Borzhomi, Tskhaltubo, Abastumani, and Pitsunda were developed because of their rich mineral springs. The springs and therapeutic mudbaths are thronged each year with the numerous guests of the sanitoria, rest homes, and retirement homes.

The profound demographic shifts characteristic of the 20th century, together with the growth of the population of our planet, have caused a quite considerable "aging of the population." This increase in the upper age brackets is largely the result of the improved standard of living, the advances of medical science, and the lowering of the mortality in the older age groups.

The demographic profile not only in Europe, but possibly also of the entire world, as E. Rosset writes, has changed and continues "to change under the influence of the aging process of the population" (Rosset, 1968, p. 229). Every year the population of our planet increases by 65 million persons, and there is every likelihood that such increases will continue.

In the USSR there are more persons 100 years of age and older than in any other country of the world. For the past 2 centuries, cases of extreme longevity have been recorded. Within a 7-year period (1798–1805), 2,084 men were counted who died at the age of 100 years and older.

Ch. Hufeland reported that in Russia, in 1801, 2,309 persons died between the ages of 90 and 130. In only 1 year, 1804, reports of deaths indicated that 1,145 persons aged 95–100 years died, 158 aged 100–105, 90 aged 105–110, 34 aged 110–115, 36 aged 115–120, 15 aged 120–125, 5 aged 125–130, and one in the 145- to 150-year age group.

I. R. Tarkhnishvili reports on the census of the population in Russia in 1819, according to which there were 1,789 centenarians in the country, two of whom had reached the age of 160 years. In 1839, while the population for European Russia (excluding the Caucasus) was 60 million, there were 1,228 cases of death of persons of advanced age, some of whom had reached the age of 160–165 years.

According to Tarkhnishvili, Russia during those years "glorified in its centenarians and exceeded by 5–6 times the number of old people in the other countries of Europe," and this despite the fact "that violent death from diseases has never taken such a tremendous sacrifice in Europe as in Russia. . . ." (Tarkhnishvili, 1891)

According to the population census of 1897, within the borders of the former Russian Empire there were 15,577 centenarians; in 1926, 29,564. These figures, however, are open to question as no rechecking was done.

According to the data of the All-Union Population Census of the USSR in 1970, the population of the Georgian SSR had increased from 4,044,045 persons in 1959 to 4,686,358 in 1970 (i.e., by 12.2%). Of the population in 1897, 7.6% was reported as 60 years of age or older. This figure rose to 8.5% in 1926, 8.8% in 1939, 10.9% in 1959, and 11.8% in 1970.

The groups of persons aged 60–69 and 80–89 increased significantly. In order to estimate the level of longevity, the criterion used was the distribution of persons aged 80 years and older per 1,000 persons of the population aged 60 years and older (Sachuk, 1966, 8–19). The longevity index throughout the Georgian SSR in 1959 was equal to 139.5 (for the USSR, 86.2); in 1970 it was 142.6

According to demographic predictions, the numbers of persons of advanced age in Georgia will continue to increase in the future. According to the All-Union Population Census of the USSR of 1970, there are more than 19,300 persons in that country who are 100 years of age and older. For every 100,000 population, there are 7.9 persons who have passed the century mark.

Figure 3–1 gives some indexes on the number of persons aged 100 years and older per 100,000 population throughout the Union Republics. From Figure 3–1, it is clear that the transcaucasian republics of Azerbaijan, Georgia, and Armenia, according to the density of persons aged 100 years and older in the general population, are the epicenter of longevity, not only of the USSR, but of the entire world. According to the data of the All-Union Population Census of the USSR for 1970, in the three transcaucasian republics, there were 4,925 persons aged 100 years and older; of them 1,844 were in the Georgian SSR.

Figure 3–2 shows the distribution of persons aged 100 years and older throughout the Georgian SSR. Of the total number of 1,844 persons aged 100 years and older, 324 live in the cities of the republic, 1,520 in rural areas.

Table 3–1 gives a representation of the age–sex structure of the population aged 100 years and older as well as residence. From Table 3–1, it is apparent that the number of females of advanced age is greater than the number of longliving males in all age–sex groups.

The human organism is constantly influenced by a complex combination of environmental factors. In cases of prolonged exposure of the body to a particular environment, the organism's physiological functions undergo change, triggering a series of adaptive mechanisms that allow the organism to exist in the given environment.

In this regard an investigation of the geography of longevity—that is, the distribution of persons of advanced age in particular regions, plays a significant role in the study of longevity.

Figure 3–1. Numbers of persons aged 100 years and older per 100,000 population for all the USSR republics. (According to materials of the All-Union Population Census of the USSR, 1970.)

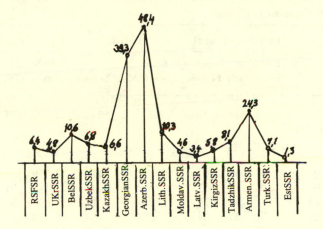

In Georgia the varied and diverse climate, along with considerable differences in geographic topography among the regions of the republic, allow some hypotheses to be made as to the effect of particular environmental factors upon life expectancy. High- and low-longevity indexes can be developed for each region, singling out favorable or

Figure 3–2. Distribution of population aged 100 years and older throughout the Georgian SSR.

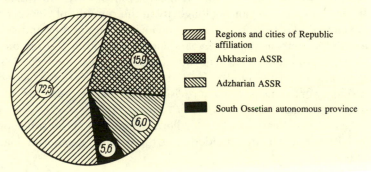

Table 3-1.

Age–sex Structure and Residence of Persons 100 Years and Older Throughout the Georgian SSR. (According to Data of the 1970 All-Union USSR Population Census).

Age	Urban and rural			Urban			Rural		
	Both Sexes	Male	Female	Both Sexes	Male	Female	Both Sexes	Male	Female
100 years and older	1,844	614	1,230	324	79	245	1,520	535	985
Of these:									
100–104	1,294	430	864	235	60	175	1,059	370	689
105–109	320	105	215	53	11	42	267	94	173
110–114	114	39	75	19	3	16	95	36	59
115–119	54	20	34	5	2	3	49	18	31
120+	62	20	42	12	3	9	50	17	33

unfavorable elements. Of course, one must bear in mind the effects of socioeconomic conditions, cultural characteristics, housing and living conditions, and life-styles. Such a medicogeographic study could introduce new foci, allowing the identification of new zones of longevity.

The problem of health-care delivery within such a diverse geographic and climatic area has not been discussed in the literature dealing with the distribution of longliving persons over the territory. In 1955, a map of regions of longevity in the republic of Georgia was developed. This map gave some idea as to the number and sex of longliving persons aged 90 years and older within the regions of Georgia. Additional materials drawn from the All-Union 1959 USSR Population Census, and the Institute for Geography of the Georgian Academy of Sciences, led to a revision of the map, which was subsequently published in the Atlas of Georgia (1965).

Georgia is situated on the northern boundaries of the subtropics, and its territories are divided into three basic geomorphological regions:

1. The southern slopes of the Major Caucasian range (elevation as high as 3,000–4,500 meters above sea level)
2. The southerly located southern Georgian mountain region (elevation 2,500–3,000 meters above sea level)
3. The zone of interalpine depressions lying between the two mountain regions. The zone on the west extends from the Black Sea east to the semideserts of Azerbaijan. The elevation here is 50–500 meters, with a maximum rise in elevation over the different territories of up to 800–900 meters above sea level.

Georgia is divided into an eastern part with a dry and continental climate, and a western part with a moist climate.

More than two-thirds of the population of the republic live in the lowlands, which cover no more than 15% to 20% of the territory of the republic. This is primarily an industrial area. One-third of the population lives in the piedmont slopes of the Caucasian range and the South Georgian mountain region. The alpine regions are sparsely populated.

The data on the average population density of Georgia as a function of elevation appears below (according to A. N. Dzhavakhishvili, 1963, p. 55):

From 0 to 500 meters	per sq. km.	83 persons
500–1,000 meters	per sq. km.	42 persons
1,000–1,500 meters	per sq. km.	19 persons
1,500–2,000 meters	per sq. km.	11 persons
Above 2,000 meters	per sq. km.	1 person

From the data, it is apparent that with increasing elevation, the population density declines sharply, and at elevations of 1,500–2,000 meters above sea level, it approaches 1. Naturally, in these zones, there are fewer longliving persons.

The territorial distribution of the population should also be examined as a further indication of the numbers of longliving persons with respect to the total population. It was found that in the high alpine regions of the republic (the southern slopes of the Caucasian range and the South Georgian mountain region), with elevations of

1,700 meters above sea level and higher, there are fewer longliving persons.

A study of the distribution of longliving persons throughout the territory of Georgia has lead to the identification of three zones of longevity. Figure 3–3 groups the different regions of the republic according to the numbers of longliving persons present. About 85% of the longliving inhabitants reside in rural districts, within the central band ranging from 500 to 1,300–1,500 meters above sea level.

Figure 3–3. Zones of Longevity in the Georgian SSR.

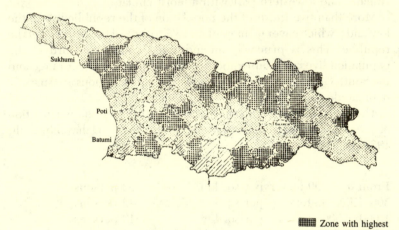

Index of longevity level for all regions (number of persons aged 90 years and older per 1,000 persons of the population aged 60 years and older)

▓▓▓ Zone with highest level of longevity
▒▒▒ Zone with relatively high level of longevity
▨▨▨ Zone with relatively low level of longevity

Many of the longliving persons are found in western Georgia, which has a moist subtropical climate, an abundance of solar radiation rich in ultraviolet rays, and other factors that favorably influence life expectancy. The distribution of longliving persons is especially high in the health resort zones, which are rich in therapeutic mineral springs.

It appears that spending one's entire life in one and the same locality, which leads to acclimatization of the organism, along with physical activity that involves repeating lifting, promotes a toughness and greater tolerance to hypoxic states. One cannot ignore, however, the beneficial effect on the organism of the mountain sunlight, which is rich in ultraviolet rays and aeroionization—both of which favor longevity.

In regions such as Tskhaltubo, Sachkher, Gulripsch, Lagodekh, Zugdid Khuloy, and others, can be found 30 or more persons who have reached the age of 100 or beyond. In the regions of Abkhazia, the Gal and Gudaut provinces, the number of persons 100 and older increases to 90. There are also isolated regions in eastern Georgia (e.g., the Goriya, Volnis, Gurdzhaan, Dmanis, and Marneul) where the number of persons 100 years and older exceeds 40. Individual regions located in the low-lying territories also contain high numbers of longliving persons. Therefore, it appears that no one single factor such as elevation determines longevity. It is rather the effect of a complex set of climatogeographic, socioeconomic, and cultural factors.

Because of the extreme variations in climatic conditions to be found within territories throughout Georgia, combinations of positive and negative environmental factors exist that can exert favorable or unfavorable influences on the life expectancy of the population. Among the important negative factors, clearly, is the elevated level of natural radiation present in the area.

4

Extraordinary Longevity in Contemporary Society

Actual human life expectancy provides a way of determining what is called, in demographics, the average life expectancy. This parameter is calculated on the basis of mortality tables. The total number of years lived by the total population born at a particular time is divided by the number of that population. In other words, the average life expectancy indicates the total number of years a given generation can be expected to live if one assumes that for the entire life span of this generation, as it passed from one age to the next, the mortality will be equal to the age-specific mortality of the year used as the basis of calculation (B. Urlanis, 1963).

Besides the average life expectancy, the French gerontologist F. Bourlier defines the life span as the maximum duration of human life—the limit "imposed on the organism by its biological characteristics and hereditary potential" (Bourlier, 1962, p. 12). The term modal life expectancy refers to the age at which the largest number dies.

According to archaeological excavations and studies of the remains of our remote ancestors, the average life expectancy in ancient times was extremely low. In the Stone Age and Bronze Age, it did not exceed 18 years. In ancient Rome, the average life expectancy was calculated as 23 years. In the Middle Ages, it fluctuated between 20 and 30 years. According to Egyptian and Roman data, Dublin and Lotka calculated the average life expectancy (at birth) and found that for the periods before our era, it was equal to 20–30 years (1936).

Dublin concluded that in the 17th and 18th centuries, the average life expectancy in the leading European countries increased by 4 years per century. For the first three-fourths of the 19th century the average life expectancy in Europe increased by 9 years, as calculated per century. In the last quarter of the 19th century, the rate of increase in Europe rose to 17 years per century (i.e., 4½ years in 25 years).

In old Russia, the average life expectancy was the lowest in Europe. Russian statisticians—the author of the mortality tables— reported short life spans. The mortality tables by which the average life expectancy was determined were first compiled by K. F. German (1819). As reported in *Narodnoye Bogatsvo*, in March 1863, in the city of St. Petersburg, official reports of the Committee of Public Health stated that the average life expectancy barely reached 16 years.

A more accurate picture of the average life expectancy of the population by the end of the 19th century was given by the mortality table compiled by S. Novoselskiy for the entire population of Russia on the basis of the 1897 census. According to these data, the average life expectancy for those born in 1896–1897 was 32–34 years (males 31–32, females 33–41).

On the basis of the 1926 census, the average life expectancy had increased: by 10.5 years for males and 13.4 for females (Kurkin, 1961, p. 347).

	Males	Females
RSFSR	40.2	45.6
UKrSSR	45.2	48.8
BelSSr	50.8	54.3
USSR	41.9	46.8

During the same period, the average life expectancy for both sexes was far higher in the rest of Europe. For example, in Sweden the average life expectancy was 52, in France 47, in England 46, and in Italy 42.

Here one should note that I. R. Tarkhnishvili in his opus *Longevity in Animals, Plants and Humans* (1891) accurately explained by sophisticated statistical methods precisely what average life expectancy means, and provided appropriate data and a method for its computation. He emphasized the importance of compiling mortality tables with population mortality indexes for separate age groups, the survival rate, and the average life expectancy.

Tarkhnishvili wrote:

All phenomena concerning life expectancy—to wit, average life span or actual and probable life expectancy at various age levels—are closely linked to mortality rates of the total population and its particular age group composition. The lower the mortality rate, the higher the average and probable life expectancy will be. (1891, p. 150).

The same is true concerning actual life expectancy.

The life expectancy of human beings is conditioned by interrelated endogenous and exogenous factors. On the biological level its basis is the genetic structure of the organism, which determines the biological time limit. The social aspect includes a wide variety of environmental factors that impinge upon humankind.

The profound social changes that took place in the USSR since the Great October Socialistic Revolution—the great economic progress; the rise in the standard of living and the cultural level of the people; the advances in public health, which lowered the mortality rate, particularly among children—all contributed to the increase in the average life expectancy of the population of the USSR. Because of the high birth rate and low mortality rate in the USSR, the population in the USSR is increasing at a higher rate than in other nations.

The Secretary General of the Central Committee of the Soviet Communist Party, Comrade L. T. Brezhnev, at a joint session of the Central Committee of the Communist Party, the Supreme Soviet of the USSR, the Supreme Soviet of the RSFSR, celebrating the 50th Anniversary of the Great October Socialistic Revolution, stated:

One can estimate the living conditions of the people by many parameters. One of the most important is human life expectancy. In old Russia, a man lived an average of 32 years. Now, among us, the average life expectancy reaches 70 years—one of the highest indexes in the world.

Only 2 years separate the indexes of the Soviet Union from the indexes of the Netherlands, where presently, women have the highest average life expectancy. One must bear in mind that it is difficult to compare a country with 12 million inhabitants (the Netherlands) with a country that numbers more than 250 million inhabitants.

As a result of such great social changes the average life expectancy in socialist countries has risen considerably. In 1921–1925, in Bulgaria, the average life expectancy did not exceed 44.6 years (44.3 years for males and 45 years for females); then in 1965–1967, it reached 70.7 years (66.8 years for males and 72.7 years for females). In the Hungarian Peoples' Republic, the average life expectancy for males in 1964 was 67 years, for females 71.8 years, whereas in 1930–1931 it was 48.7 and 58.2 years, respectively. In Czechoslovakia, there is a decided increase in the average life expectancy. In 1967, this index for males was 67.7, for females 73.7 years. At the beginning of the century, the average life expectancy in Germany for males was 41 years, and for females 44 years. Now, in the German Democratic Republic, it has reached 70 years for males and almost 75 years for females.

Table 4–1.

Average Life Expectancy of the USSR Population and That of Prerevolutionary Russia.[a]

| Years | Average life expectancy | | |
	Both sexes	Males	Females
1896–1897	32	31	33
1926–1927	44	42	47
1958–1959	69	64	72
1963–1964	70	66	74

[a]D. F. Chebotarev. *Dolgoletive (Longevity)*. Moscow, 1970, p. 18.

A further increase in the average life expectancy could be anticipated through a reduction in mortality throughout the life span, particularly during childhood. Such a reduction could be achieved through improvements in public health service and upgrading of the general standard of living.

Although, as Table 4–2 indicates, the average life expectancy has increased significantly among developed nations, the average life expectancy in underdeveloped countries is extremely low.

Accurate demographic information is imperative for studying population shifts, for developing statistics on longevity, and for organizing medical assistance. Knowledge of exact calendar age is necessary in a number of cases in order to solve a number of problems involving medicolegal and occupational health issues. In such instances, it is important that individuals, especially those of advanced age, know their exact age.

Many researchers have indicated that elderly persons are prone to exaggerating their age. Such exaggeration of one's age is common even among well-educated older persons. Consequently, census data cannot be totally relied on for determining the size of an elderly age group within the population (See I. R. Tarkhnishvili, Z. G. Frenkel, U. A. Spasokukotskiy, G. Z. Pitskhelauri, N. N. Sachuk, R. D. Alikishiev, and others).

Even I. R. Tarkhnishvili, when determining the age of longliving persons, warned of the possibility of obtaining erroneous data. He wrote:

> Information relative to the exact age of extremely old men who are found in one country or another should be confirmed on the basis of documentary data, i.e., should be checked by birth certificates or other reliable attested information related to the various circumstances of life. When gathering such information, one should not be guided at all by oral statements of the old people themselves, who, because of forgetfulness, or coquettishness peculiar to this age group, brag about their old age. Some may add to the number of years lived, and 90–95 year-olds become centenarians for the census. Such fabrications have often led statisticians into great errors. . . . (Tarkhnishvili, 1891, p. 136)

According to the oldest statistical data, the number of centenarians

Table 4–2.

Data on Average Life Expectancy in Selected Countries

Country	Average life expectancy[a]		Percentage of population by age groups in 1970[b]		
	Males	Females	Under 14 yr.	15–64 yr.	over 65 yr.
Austria (1969)	66.4	73.3	25	61	14
Belgium (1959–1963)	67.7	73.3	24	63	13
Gabon (1960–1961)	25.0	45.0	33	61	6
India (1951–1960)	41.9	40.6	42	55	3
Indonesia (1960)	47.5	47.5	45	53	2
Spain (1960)	67.3	71.9	28	63	9
Italy (1960–1962)	67.2	72.3	25	64	11
Canada (1965–1967)	68.8	75.2	31	61	8
Netherlands (1968)	71.0	76.4	27	63	10
Pakistan (1962)	53.7	48.8	47	50	3
Peru (1960–1965)	52.6	55.5	45	52	3
Portugal (1959–1962)	60.7	66.4	29	62	9
Togo (1961)	31.6	38.5	45	53	2
France (1968)	68.0	75.5	25	62	13
W. Germany (1966–1968)	67.6	73.6	24	63	13
Central African Republic 1959–1963	33.3	36.0	42	55	3
Chad (1963–1964)	29.0	35.0	45	53	2
Chile (1960–1961)	54.4	60.0	39	56	5
Switzerland (1958–1963)	68.7	74.1	24	65	11
Yugoslavia (1966–1967)	64.7	69.0	28	65	7

[a]Source: United Nations. *Demographic Reference Book*. 1970. In parentheses: the time when the study was conducted.
[b]Source: Division of ethnic population of the UNO, calculated increase in population by age, sex, region, and country, 1965–1985, average values.

in Bavaria in the 1871 census was 27, but a recheck showed that 15 of them had not even reached 90 years, and only one widow was older than 100. In Bulgaria, according to the 1920 census, there were 2,161 persons older than 100 years. After a careful check of the 1926 census, their number did not exceed 1,756. A special examination of 100-year-old persons in the places that indicated this age on the census sheet revealed that the number of centenarians was no greater than 158—11 times less than recorded by the census. In this instance, none was older than 112, whereas according to the first census, there were 38 such people, including six who were 120 and four who were 125.

Such a rechecking of persons 100 years old and older was also conducted in Italy. According to the Italian 1921 census, there were 256 persons of both sexes 100 years of age. In 1926, the Italian Statistical Institute rechecked the data on these persons for the purpose of establishing causes and rates of mortality. The check showed that only 51 were actually older than 100 during the period of the 1921 census—five times less than the number of centenarians originally registered.

In Russia, a checking of documents of centenarians appearing in the 1897 census showed that the number of centenarians was exaggerated by five times. In the All-Union 1959 Census of the USSR Population, there were 28,015 persons 100 years old and older, but a check of documents reduced this figure to 21,708.

Recognizing the importance of establishing the accurate age of longliving persons, the Institute of Gerontology of the USSR Academy of Medical Sciences included rechecking and documentation of age in its program of medical examinations of selected persons 80 years and older. According to the method used, the year of birth is ascertained by a systematic comparison of all entries on the chart dealing with birth year and age. The information on birth certificates is taken under consideration, as well as the passport, village council accounting books, and other documents. These data (besides birth certificates) are compared with the questionnaire data and other questions on the chart where age and year are shown.

When determining age, the subject or closest relatives are closely questioned. Information gained from such interviews are correlated with events of historical, local, and familial significance.

N. N. Sachuk, in her studies on the accuracy of the calendar age of persons 80 years old and older who participated in a research project of the Institute of Gerontology and Experimental Pathology of the USSR Academy of Medical Sciences, found significant inaccuracies in statements with respect to calendar age. Such inaccuracies were true of men and women, and of both rural and urban residents.

In order to ascertain calendar age, a study was developed to test the accuracy of the age statements made by 704 longliving persons aged 100 years and older. In the reexamination, data on age and year of birth, as indicated on birth certificates, passports, village council accounting books, and other documents were double-checked and compared.

The age of the longliving person was compared with the ages of children, grandchildren, and great-grandchildren. These data were verified by asking such control questions as: At what age and in what year did the longliving person get married; when were the first and last child born; and other questions related to some significant event particular to the locality where the longliving person resided.

It was found that of 704 persons, 665 (94.5%) were 100 years of age and older. The age of 39 of the longliving persons (5.5%) was less than 100 years, and that the age of 134 persons (19%) actually did not coincide with the data of the census but was within the limits of 100 years and older. In general, there was lack of correspondence between actual age and the statement in the census for 173 longliving persons (24.5%).

In 565 cases, the documented age coincided with the birth certificates, passport, or village council accounting book, and in 122 cases it did not correspond to the documents. Correspondence between age and passport data was found in 234 cases. Since the longliving persons of Georgia received passports after 1932, when already mature and even old, this precluded their falsifying their age.

A symposium held in Leningrad in June 1962 had great significance for the development of a classification and nomenclature appropriate for the periods of aging and a rationale for establishing age boundaries. Age boundaries were agreed upon establishing that persons 60–74 years of age are *mature*, those 75–89 years of age are *old*, and those 90 years old and older are *longliving*. Such a chronological grouping of the periods of aging was also accepted at a meeting of the World Health Organization in May 1963 in Kiev.

Throughout history one can find numerous examples of persons having lived for extraordinarily long periods of time. Some examples appear below.

Contigern (San Mungo), the founder of the bishopric of Glasgow, and Ktsarten Petrark both lived to 185. The latter was so alert that up until the last few days before his death, he continued to walk through the streets with his cane. His oldest son was 155 and his youngest 97.

The Englishman Thomas Parr was presented to the king in London at the age of 152 as a rare case of longevity. He died on November 15, 1635 and was buried in Westminister Abbey. (For more details, see Pitskhelauri, 1963.)

Queen Victoria sent her portrait to the aged postal clerk Robert Taylor with the inscription: "A gift from Queen Victoria to R. Taylor in honor of his great and unparalleled old age." This gift so excited the old man he died 3 months later at the age of 134.

The Iranian Saied Abutalem Musavi, who lived in the little village of Bak Adan, 550 miles south of Teheran, had lived to 191 at this writing. This longliving person is the head of a tribe consisting of several hundreds of his grandsons, great-grandsons, and great-great-grandsons. His fifth wife is 105.

At the end of March 1958, in the city of Bogotá (Colombia), J. Perriera died at the age of 169. He was born in 1789 and participated in the struggle for the independence of Colombia.

In the Syrian town of Mzaz, 163-year-old Makhmud Vardan died in 1963. He was considered to be the oldest man in Syria.

According to the agency France Press, in January 1966, in the city of Casablanca, the Moroccan Hadj Mahommed Ben Bashir died at the age of 166. He had 35 sons and daughters and 152 grandchildren.

In one of the settlements not far from the capital of the Ivory Coast lives 162-year-old Musse Wattara. This longliving person does not complain of ill health and even travels to other countries. He has 13 children and many grandchildren and great-grandchildren. His family has grown to such an extent that direct descendents of the old man can be found in many of the countries of West Africa.

During the All-Union Population Census of the USSR in 1959, the following record cases of longevity were discovered.

Aytraliyev Ismail, 160 years old (Azerbaijan SSR, Georgian region, village of Atrallar); Mertiyeva Sarguz Kerem, 156 years old (Azerbaijan SSR, Masalin region, village of Shikhlar); Chernyshev Ivan, 151 years old (Kazakh SSR, Alma-Ata).

The oldest man in Soviet Azerbaijan and in the USSR was considered to be the recently deceased peasant of the village of Barzavu, Shirali Mislimov. At the time when the Hulistan treaty was concluded with Persia in 1813, which made Azerbaijan part of Russia, he was 8 years old. At the age of 168, he was alert and even worked a little. The number of his descendents has reached 220.

In the village of Pirassura of the Azerbaijan SSR, Makhmud Eyvazov, founder of the collective Komsomol farm, lived for 150 years. His health and mental alertness were remarkable.

At the present time in the settlement of Tikyaband in Azerbaijan lives the oldest resident of that republic, collective farmer Medzhid Agayev, who is 139 years old. His family consists of 150 children, grandchildren, great-grandchildren, and great-great-grandchildren. When he reached the age 136, the administration of the collective farm forbade him to walk with the flock and assigned him a quieter job: herding cows.

Much attention has been centered upon the longliving persons who were found in Georgia during the All-Union Population Census of 1970: R. V. Gogoladze, 132 years old (Lagodekh region, village of Shroma); L. G. Pukhashivili, 130 years old (Karel's region, village of Bani); M. D. Mushkundiani, 129 years old (Tsager region, village of Chkhuteli); L. G. Bigvava, 130 years old (Gal region, village of Ganatleba), and others.

A resident of the village of Yermani (South Ossetian autonomous province), Ye. P. Koroyev, had survived to the age of 156. Until the end of his life, he was distinguished by his mental alertness, his good memory, and his work as a fieldhand.

The Abkhazian, Khapara Kiut (1785–1935), lived to be 155 years old.

In the Ochamchir region, Zhats Kiut worked in the village of Kindgi until he reached the age of 144. He participated actively in developing the orchards of the collective farm. His brother Mamsyr Kiut died in 1946 at the age of 149.

Ashkhanger Bzhaniya lived to the age of 148. A portrait of him as a person representing exceptional longevity was hung in the Dresden Museum.

In the village of Gentsvishi (Svanetiya) lives Daday Chopliani, age 129. He had been witness to the radical changes in the life of the Svans in the second half of the 19th century.

The recently deceased collective farmer of the village of Lykhny, A. Kh. Piliya, was 122. He was distinguished throughout his life by his tremendous working capacity.

In the village of Atara of Ochamchir region lives Selakh Butba, who is 121 years old. He is the father of a very large family. Many old men who have passed the century mark live in the Lentekh region. One resident of the village of Lausheri, Saba Babliani, has reached the age of 119, and is still mentally alert.

G. Khvinchianshvili, a resident of the village of Meore-Sviri, is 116. He participated in the struggle of the Bulgarian people against the Ottoman yolk in 1878 and remembers the events of those days clearly.

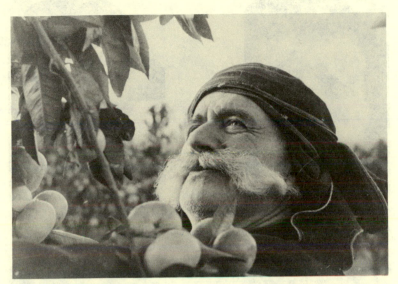

Plate 1. Georgian SSR. I. Menunargia, one of the oldest fruit pickers in a citrus fruit collective.

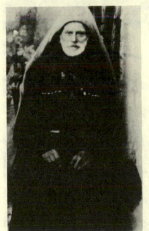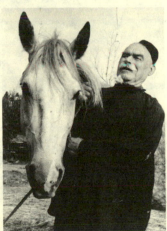

Plate 2. Georgian SSR. D. Ch. Labachuya, who died at the age of 142.

Plate 3. Georgian SSR. I. Dzavachishivili of the city of Tbilisi. A great lover of horses who was born in 1866.

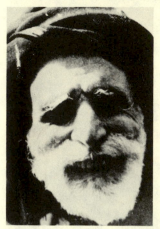
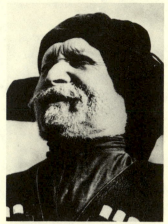

Plate 4.   Georgian SSR. Sulaman Arshba, 123 years old.
Plate 5.   Georgian SSR. A. Piliya, 120 years old.

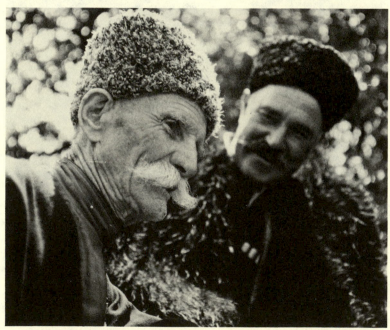

Plate 6.   Old friends from the collective farm Lihni/Abkhasia. On the left is Temur Vanacha, 110 years old, and on the right, K. Dzhidzhariya, 75 years old.

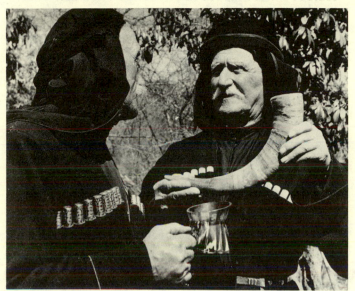

Plate 7.   A. Shlarba and T. Sharmat from Abkhasia who passed the 100 mark some time ago.

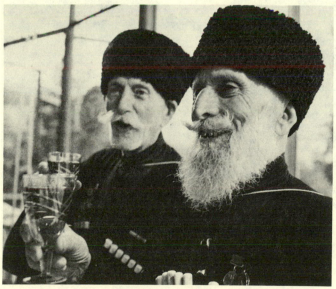

Plate 8.   Centenarian collective farmers: A. Gegechkori and O. Mkhedzhe from the Zhestafonskovo region of Georgia.

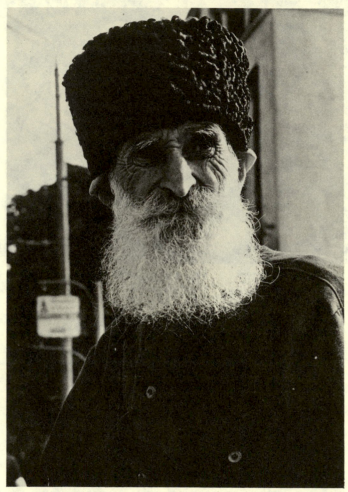

Plate 9.   A. Gabadadzhe at 92 years of age is the oldest collective farmer of the village of Gurna in the Tkvibulskovo region of Georgia.

5

Women and Longevity

The life expectancy of women in most countries of the world is higher than that of men. This is the case even when one takes into consideration the claiming of younger ages by women and the fact that older men display a form of "coquettishness" by exaggerating their age.

In the USSR, as well as in other economically developed countries of the world, longevity is higher among women than among men, a fact explained by the high mortality among men in all age groups. According to the data of the 1970 United Nations *Demographic Reference Book,* the average life expectancy of women in Sweden is somewhat more than 75 years; in the Netherlands, Switzerland, and Norway about 75 years; in France 74; in Denmark, the United States, Czechoslovakia, and New Zealand 73–74 years. The life expectancy of the women of Iceland is high—76 years; that of Japan 72–75; and Puerto Rico 71–88. Among the African countries, the lowest life expectancy for women is found in Guinea at 26; in the Upper Volta, it is 31.1.

However, there are countries such as Sri Lanka, Pakistan, Cambodia, and Guatemala where men live longer than women; while in Bolivia the life expectancy is the same for both sexes. India has always been a country where the life expectancy of men is higher than that of women, because of the high maternal mortality and the harsh living conditions. Extremely early marriage, usually after the age of 12, has strongly undermined the health of the women. In recent times, however, the life expectancy of women has increased significantly.

An indicator of the level of mortality, as is known, is the average life expectancy. For men in the USSR, the average life expectancy is 66 years, while for women it is 74. The reduction of the discrepancy of 8 years would greatly enhance the lives of both sexes.

In the table below are listed the numbers of males and females who have reached the age of 80 and older within the population of persons aged 60 years and older throughout the Union Republics of the USSR (per 1,000 persons according to materials of the 1959 All-Union Census ["World Population Reference Manual," 1965, p. 131]).

The upper limit of both male and female population aged 80 years

	Males	Females
USSR	78	98
RSFSR	77	97
Ukrainian SSR	68	90
Belorussian SSR	83	108
Uzbek SSR	73	85
Kazakh SSR	76	91
Georgian SSR	134	144
Azerbaijan SSR	144	173
Lithuanian SSR	81	118
Moldavian SSR	62	75
Latvian SSR	102	128
Kirgiz SSR	85	91
Tadzhik SSR	68	84
Armenian SSR	121	141
Turkmenian SSR	76	90
Estonian SSR	84	114

and older is found in the transcaucasian republics. Females predominate in these age groups.

The greater life expectancy of females compared to males in Russia and the USSR is clearly illustrated by Table 5–1.

The predominance of females aged 100 years and older over the number of males of these ages is clear according to the data of the 1959 All-Union Population Census of the USSR, in which of the total number of longliving persons (21,708), there were 16,276 females and only 5,432 males. For 100,000 inhabitants, there are 6 males of these ages and 14 females. The predominance of females over males is also noted in all age groups up to 120 years and older.

Thus, of the total number of 1,357 longliving persons aged 100–114, there are 407 males and 950 females. Of 578 persons aged 120 and older, 219 are males and 359 females, and so on.

In the Georgian SSR, as stated above, of 1,844 persons aged 100 and older, there were 1,230 females and 614 males. The predominance of females is notable in all age groups.

In the 100–104 age group, there were 864 females and 430 males; 215 and 105 in the 105–109 group; 75 and 39 in the 110–114 group; 34

TABLE 5–1

Average Life Expectancy of Males as Compared to Females in the USSR[a]

Dates	Average life expectancy (yr.)		No. of yrs. female life expectancy greater than men's life expectancy
	Males	Females	
1896–1897	31	33	2
1926–1927	42	47	5
1954–1955	61	67	6
1955–1956	63	69	6
1957–1958	64	71	7
1958–1959	64.4	71.7	7.3
1960–1961	65	73	8

[a]Source: B. Ts. Urlanis. *Birth rate and human life expectancy in the USSR*. Moscow, 1963, p. 113.

and 20 in the 115–119 group; and 42 and 20 in the group aged 120 years and older.

The differences cited in life expectancy of males and females can be explained by a number of factors. A factor of great importance is the high mortality of males due to chronic intoxication by alcohol, nicotine, and industrial pollution. Another is the high accident rate. Smoking alone is responsible for severe damage to the male organism. The mortality from malignant tumors of the respiratory organs among smoking men is six times greater than among women. No less important is the effect of wartime stresses on the viability of the male organism.

The predominance of longliving women over men—the high average life expectancy of women—can also be explained by the greater biogenetic endurance found in the female organism even in the early stages of its development. Such survival is linked to the biological mission of the female—the care of offspring. This conclusion is in agreement with the opinion of I. R. Tarkhnishvili, who wrote:

"Nature cares more for preservation of the race than prolonging the life of individuals. From this standpoint, it is understandable why females of many animal species have a longer life span than males." (Tarkhnishvili, 1891, p. 141)

The data obtained by U. A. Spasokukotskiy et al. on the longevity of women indicate that the high level of longevity of women is due to the physiological characteristics of the female organism, such as the compensatory mechanisms developed during the process of evolution in connection with the childbearing function. (pp. 33–44)

The physical endurance of women was pointed out by N. G. Chernyshevskiy in his novel *Chto delat?* "The woman's body," says the hero of the novel, Lopukhov,

more effectively withstands natural destructive forces—such as climate, weather, inadequate diet. Medicine and physiology have paid little attention to the analysis of this phenomenon, but statistics have already given an incontestable general answer: The average life expectancy of women is greater than that of men. From this, it is evident that the female organism is stronger.

N. Sachuk writes:

> That significant "leap" that women have made in surpassing men in
> longevity over a relatively short period, historically speaking, cannot be
> explained solely by the biological aspects of their organism, advantages
> which nature provided females in order to insure the preservation of the
> human race. It cannot be logically justified solely by genetic program-
> ming. In spite of our understanding of the important role of social con-
> ditioning with respect to sex differences and longevity, the effects of
> socio-biological factors on longevity have yet to be measured (Sachuk,
> 1972, pp. 339–340).

Women, therefore, should be considered the strong and not the
weak sex. Emphasizing the clear predominance in the number of
longliving women, I. R. Tarkhnishvili remarked that in women, the
characteristics of senescence appear somewhat earlier, but in comparison with men, this does not interfere with their living to an
advanced age.

A reduction in the factors causing the higher mortality among men
will allow a significant reduction in the gap between life expectancy of
men and women. M. S. Bednyy writes:

> Today, we must address the question of further increasing the life expec-
> tancy of the population—this means, above all, to direct our efforts at
> bringing its dimensions for men close to those already achieved by
> women. It is necessary to study the factors responsible for such great
> differences and to implement on a practical scale scientifically verified
> socio-hygienic measures to alter the situation in the desired direction
> (Bednyy, 1972, p. 183).

It is noteworthy that almost all of the longliving women of Georgia
are housewives who had been married for approximately 50–80
years. The benefits of family life on life expectancy is confirmed by
the data on the marital status of longliving women.

A study of data on 2,369 longliving women aged 80–100 years and
404 women 100 years and older indicated that only 1.7% of the total
number examined were not married. Among the centenarians, the
largest number of marriages took place at the age of 15 to 20.

However, cases have been noted of women marrying at the age of 11–14 (7% to 8%), and also of women marrying comparatively late, after 35 years of age. (See Figure 5–1.)

Figure 5–1. Marital status of population of Georgian SSR aged 100 years and older according to data of All-Union 1970 USSR Census (in %).

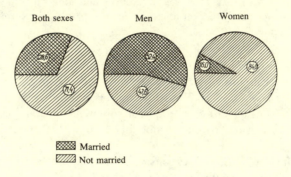

It should be noted that in the past, among the inhabitants of the Caucasus, including Georgia, cases of early marriage were recorded. Such marriages are now forbidden by Soviet law as the developing female is not considered ready for motherhood until the age of 18.

Popular opinion often regards pregnancy, childbirth, and the postnatal period as harmful to the health and longevity of women. Scientific studies, however, have shown that systematic avoidance of pregnancy and childbirth through abortion causes significant damage to the female organism.

Some women fear that pregnancy accelerates the processes of aging and the wearing out of the body. Such fears are clearly unfounded. Even I. R. Tarkhnishvili, emphasizing the great capacity of longliving persons to reproduce offspring, remarked that this was sometimes a possibility even to the last year of life.

I. F. Zhordaniya wrote:

The claims that women, unless they use contraceptives or resort to abortions, face premature aging and will be limited in their ability to productively engage in social and political life, are largely exaggerated. . . . Systematic avoidance of pregnancies and births for several years, whether conducted through the use of contraceptives, abortions, or other antiphysiological means, causes certain, and sometimes quite considerable, damage (1960, p. 10).

The fertility of women—their capacity to bear children—is one of the factors that acts favorably upon their health and longevity. Studies indicate that longliving women in the past were extremely fertile and that many preserved this function to comparatively advanced ages. Historically, throughout Georgia as a whole, of the married longliving persons who reached the age of 100 or older only about 4% were childless. For longliving persons residing in rural areas the infertility percentage equaled 4.5%; whereas among longliving persons of Tbilisi the infertility figure reached 8.8%.

A study of more than 2,700 women aged 80 to 100 years and older showed that about 80% had three or more children, while 21% had from six to nine children. In the majority of families investigated, thus, there were from four to six children. The largest number of longliving persons who have 13 children, are those who are 100 years of age and older. Individual cases of 15, 17, and 20 children have been recorded.

Listed below are data on mothers with numerous children.

In the village of Dzimiti of the Makharadze region, T. Kekeliya, 107 years old, has raised 11 children. S. Gogodze, who lived in Borzhomi, is more than 100 years old and has 11 children.

Tarasiya and Matada Pureliani of Lentekhi (Svanetiya) are both 100 years old. They have been married for 80 years and have nine children, 18 grandsons and granddaughters, 32 great-grandsons and great-granddaughters, 17 great-great-grandsons and great-great-granddaughters. This large family totals some 70 members.

G. Kapanadze of the village of Chkhirauli is 113 years old; she has eight children and 70 grandchildren and great-grandchildren. V. Mukbaniani of Lentekhi is about 100 and has nine children and 63 grandchildren.

The data presented above clearly indicate that early marriage, a high level of reproductivity ending in full-term births, and the avoidance of abortions, all contribute to strengthening the health and increasing the life expectancy of women.

History is replete with examples of unusual longevity and a high level of productivity of women in ancient times. Terencia, the wife of Cicero, lived to be 103; the Empress Livia Augusta lived to be 90 years old. Lyutenia, a well-known actress in her time, who charmed her audiences by the realism of her portrayals, embarked on a stage career in early youth, played in the theater for 100 years, and even appeared on the stage in the 112th year of her life.

Galeria Copiola, the Roman actress and danseuse, appeared on the stage 90 years after her first performance in order to surprise Pompey the Great. She was seen on the stage once more, at the crowning of Augustus.

One of the oldest women of the world was the Ossetian Tayabad Aniyeva, who lived to be 181 years old.

In 1928 the Turkish woman Fatima Khanum died at the age of 164. Today the oldest woman in Turkey is Hatice Korkmaz, who is 132 years old. In her long life, she married three times, and has suffered only two mild colds.

In March 1964, 169-year-old Hacer Issek Nine died in Ankara following a heart attack. The last words of the oldest woman of Turkey were: "I have not yet lived enough in this world."

The Frenchwoman Marie Priou, who died in 1938, lived to the age of 158, preserving a sound mind despite physical decline. During the last 10 years of her life, she subsisted exclusively on cheese and goat's milk.

Virginia Contesoise, born January 9, 1864 in Monjamel, France, celebrated the 100th anniversary of her birth by announcing to her family members: "I have lived to 100 because I worked a lot, ate only good natural food and home-baked bread, did not overindulge in meat, especially pork, and drank only water."

According to census data of 1957, the oldest resident of Moscow was L. V. Puzhak, who was born in 1803. She met Pushkin, Nekrasov, and Chekhov. At the age of 154, she still worked on a farm, did her own shopping, and prepared her own food.

Galuyeva Fatimat from the village of Gizel of the North Ossetian ASSR lived to be 128 years old. Until shortly before her death in

1960, she engaged in housework, spun, embroidered linen, knitted socks, and enjoyed a fine memory and good vision.

In the Dagestan ASSR in the settlement of Chankurbi of the Buynak region lived the oldest woman of this republic, the darghin-woman Ashura Telmekova, who died at the age of 148. At the time of the uprising in Shamil, she was married for a second time. On several occasions, she saw Shamil in person with his detachment of Myurids during their passage through the Kadar mountains.

Also in this Republic, in the mountain village of Kuha-Makli, live the three sisters Bagandova: Khamis, Khadizhat, and Khamis the Younger. The oldest sister is 116, the middle 113, and the youngest 110 years. The sisters are very diligent, prepare their own food, wash, sew, and keep house. Khamis the Younger is still working in the Kolkhoz (collective farm) bakery.

One of the oldest residents of Kirgizia, Sel ti Kuliyevoy, has celebrated her 121st birthday. She has more than 40 grandsons and great-grandsons. This longliving woman manages all her own domestic affairs, and is raising her youngest grandchildren.

Khfaf Lasurii, a resident of the village of Kvitouli of Ochamnir region of Abkhazia, is 138 years old. Despite her advanced age, she is still working in the Kolkhoz on the tea plantation.

The village of Tedeleti in the Dzhav region of Georgia is called the "village of the longliving." Its inhabitants include many people who have lived beyond 100. Recently, the people of Tedeleti celebrated the birthday of their fellow villager Liza Gadiyeva, who had reached 125. Friends, children, grandchildren, and great-grandchildren, as well as guests from the neighboring villages, came to congratulate the oldest woman of the village and to celebrate. Liza Gadiyeva does not think of herself as old; she is alert and full of energy. One of L. Gadiyeva's friends, Pena Tandelova, was 115 that year. Her family includes some 86 persons.

Not far from Tbilisi, in Digomi, live M. Zhamutashvili, who is 100 years old, and L. Kutsniashvili, 102, both of whom continue to work. In the village of Zenit of the Kobulet region, lives T. Mzhavanadze, who has reached the age of 100.

In order to maintain the health and to improve the life expectancy of women, the prevention of disease of the female reproductive organs is of singular importance. The female organism is subject to inflammatory diseases of the genitals, benign tumors of the uterus, so-called fibromyomas, menstrual disorders, and infertility. The greatest damage to the health of women is caused by malignant neoplasms, including cancer of the uterus and its adnexa.

Women's health is affected to a certain degree, in some instances, by pathologies associated with menopause. This may result in a reduction of work capacity and a highly pronounced vegetoneurosis. In such cases, the woman should consult a specialist in order to receive proper medical assistance. The studies of the I. F. Zhordaniya Research Institute on Human Generative Functions of the Ministry of Health of the Georgian SSR indicate that problems related to menopause can be prevented and successfully treated.

The sexual education of girls, which should begin in the early years, at home and in school, has great significance for the attainment of longevity. Participation in physical exercise and athletics plays an important role in controlling premature aging. Beneficial effects on the female organism and its nervous system can be derived through conditioning the body by employing such natural aids as sunbaths, air baths, and water treatments. The use of nature's gifts fortifies the female organism, raising its resistance to diseases and promoting longevity. Physical exercises are widely used in industry, as they improve the oxygen supply to the tissues and metabolism, prevent fatigue, reduce morbidity, and increase labor productivity. Physical exercises are especially recommended for women who spend much time in a sitting position, as a way of eliminating the symptoms of congestion in the region of the minor pelvis. Women who regularly engage in physical exercise, experience fewer complications during pregnancy and childbirth.

Women inclined to obesity and who are subject to the various diseases associated with overweight, should standardize their diet, sleep, work, and rest. A more regular daily routine will aid them in controlling premature aging and wrinkling. To prevent the onset of early senescence and obesity, a balanced and nutritious diet should be begun well before the appearance of even slight signs of aging. Overeating, especially excessive consumption of animal fats, promotes the development of atherosclerosis, hypertension, and gout.

Many opportunities are available for the preservation of health and the prevention of premature aging. Medical treatment, however, should be properly combined with general hygienic measures. No medication will be effective unless the woman's life-style, as well as her determination and unremitting efforts, are directed toward the preservation of her youth.

Our studies have shown that every woman can retard the aging process. She must, however, pay strict attention to the rules that help control premature aging. Such rules include the following: guard and strengthen the nervous system, preserving its high tonus; work without becoming overfatigued, maintaining a balance between periods of work and rest; strictly observe the rules of personal hygiene—sexual hygiene in particular.

All of the above, as well as physical exercise, proper diet, adequate sleep and toughening of the body will aid every woman in preventing premature aging and prolonging life.

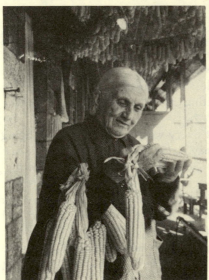
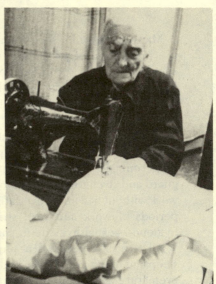

Plate 10. Georgian SSR. O. M. Kashibadze, 107 years old, resident of the city of Batum (Adzhar Republic). An able-bodied worker, she enjoys tending her personal plot on the collective farm.
Plate 11. Georgian SSR. Seamstress Salome Dolidze, 103 years old.

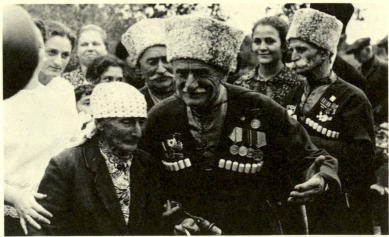

Plate 12. The longliving, D. Aiba, 85 years old, (on the right) and L. Khfaf, 138 years old (on the left), visiting with collective farmers of the village.

6

Life-Styles
of the Old
and Longliving

In contemporary gerontological literature, much attention is devoted to the physiology and pathology of aging, and the clinical aspects of these largely biomedical problems. Less attention is paid to questions related to the effect of the external environment on physical states, even though environmental factors play the leading role in determining the aging process, as well as longevity. Comparatively few studies deal specifically with areas such as life-style, standard of living, and health status of longliving persons.

The concept of life-style must, of necessity, include material and spiritual aspects—the family, general living conditions, diet, the daily routine, customs and habits of the total population, rest and leisure, health care, as well as societal expectations.

In Georgia, in collaboration with A. Agadzhanova, a sample of 6,226 persons within the categories of the old and longliving were studied to gauge the effects of life-style upon life expectancy. Of these, 626 were 100–130 years of age, and resided in all parts of the Republic; 5,054 were from 80–99 years of age and lived in the rural regions of the Republic; and 546 were 80–99 years of age and lived in Tbilisi. Factors considered were: age, sex, national background, education, residence, financial status, health care, sources of income, role within the family, marital status, work role, and diet.

Considering the fact that older persons tend to exaggerate their age, the accuracy of the actual age of subjects was established according to specific laboratory methods routinely practiced in the Tbilisi Gerontology Center.

Residential data on the persons studied indicated that the majority resided in rural areas, a few in regional centers, and only very few in the cities of the republic.

The majority of the longliving residents of Tbilisi (59%) had been village laborers who had migrated to the city. Of the total number studied, 23.3% had moved to the city while young (20–30 years), 14.5% when middle-aged, and 16% after the age of 50. The reduced migration after the age of 50 years and older can be attributed to persons' settling down to a particular life-style when reaching the categories of the mature and old. This can be regarded as a form of adaptation to the environment.

A study of the housing conditions of longliving persons of the rural regions of Georgia showed that about 97% of them lived in good or satisfactory housing. The longliving shared with other family members spacious, airy houses consisting of four to six rooms with a veranda (ayvani) and a yard. About 26% of the longliving resided in their own homes, 70% with the families of their children; others were found in residential homes for the elderly or nursing homes.

The majority of the rural longliving, had a private room of adequate size that satisfied hygienic requirements. In the yards are found gardens, orchards, and vineyards. The environment is clean and neat, including the living quarters and yard.

In evaluating the adequacy of housing conditions of the longliving residents of Tbilisi, it was found that 92.5% of them live in good or satisfactory apartments. Those whose housing was regarded as poor, were primarily persons who did not want to live with family members; those who lived in isolated regions with only poor housing available; or single individuals who had never married and had no living relatives.

All of the subjects received some form of income. Pensions were received by 17% of the longliving persons of the rural districts, while a significant number received funds from the Kolkhoz administration. The greater part of the financial support in old age was donated by children, grandchildren, and great-grandchildren. About 26.3% of the longliving lived with their own families in their own households, 70% in the households of their children, and only 3.7% lived alone. Among the longliving of Tbilisi, there are 75.1% pensioners.

FAMILY LIFE

Of the total number of persons studied in Tbilisi, 25.1% lived with their spouses, 64.4% with the families of their children, and only 10.5% were single.

Living with family members who are solicitous and who provide appropriate care is one factor that has a positive effect upon life expectancy. Ch. Hufeland once noted that all people who survived to advanced age were married. Some had been married several times. No bachelor has been recorded to have lived to 100. I. R. Tarkhnishvili also wrote: "Married life, beginning at the 20th year, represents a more favorable condition for sustaining life and provides greater life enhancement than does the unmarried state." (Tarkhnishvili, 1891, p. 101)

The positive effect of family life upon life expectancy is confirmed by data on marital status. Among the longliving, cases of late marriages, when longliving men married younger women, have resulted in marriages that have lasted as long as 80–100 years or more. Among 626 subjects aged 100 years and older, only two men and eight women were not married.

Out of 5,054 subjects in the two categories of old persons and longliving individuals from rural districts, 2% were unmarried. Among the longliving of Tbilisi, only 3.9% were unmarried.

The data of life expectancy and marital status of the longliving present interesting material for speculation. Within the group aged 100 and above, 56.5% had been married from 50 to 80 years; 10.9% had been married for 80–90 years; and 3%, 90 years and longer. It appears that marriages of long duration have a positive effect upon life expectancy. The family, which combines in itself individual and group origins, is a link that binds not only the biological and social aspects of human life, but also the public life as well. Certainly marriage normalizes the sex life.

PHYSICAL ACTIVITY

Physical activity is considered by the longliving to be indispensable to long life. Those who live in alpine regions referred to regular climbs and descents as toughening the body and assisting in adaptation to climatic conditions. About 64% of the longliving travel independently within their own city or village, and engage in travel of some distance. Physical activity as part of a total life-style, particularly to offset obesity, is characteristic of the longliving of Georgia, Dagestan, Checheno-Ingushetia, and other republics.

More than 60% of persons living to 100 years or older are self-sufficient. About 80% of the men and 68% of the women aged 80 years and older, out of the total of those who do not work in Kolkhozes and Sovkhozes (state farms), are engaged in housework, garden, or look after livestock and poultry. Many continue to enjoy hunting and riding horseback.

The longliving are early risers who go to bed no later than 8 or 9 P.M., and sleep deeply for up to 10 hours. During 7 or 8 months of the year, many sleep outdoors; only during the winter do they sleep indoors.

The longliving of Georgia spend almost the entire day in natural settings, in fresh clean air, in an environment saturated with ultraviolet rays. They do not have to squeeze into buses or to force their way through crowds. The absence of hurrying, the peaceful village life, orderly planned work and leisure time—all allow the Georgians to live to advanced years.

The longliving usually observe strict personal hygiene; this is the fundamental basis of their mode of life. They bathe frequently, keep their bodies clean, and wear clean clothing. Among the longliving of Dagestan, Checheno-Ingushetia, and Azerbaijan, the use of bathing after elimination has been made into a ritual. The careful personal hygiene of the longliving of the Caucasus helps prevent disease and contributes to their long life.

EDUCATIONAL LEVELS

The longliving also use their leisure time profitably. They listen to the radio, read, or watch television. They actively participate in social life and creative activities. A sustained interest in life, and continuous communication with the mainstream of life, are important indices of normal psychological health among the longliving. Generally, the longliving from villages are little read or totally illiterate, whereas among the urban population, one encounters persons who have completed an intermediate and even a higher education.

It is commonly recognized that an active intellectual life in youth is preserved well into retirement and even into advanced age. This is particularly true of urban populations. Such capability, however, is preserved as long as the person maintains intellectual interests and actively utilizes his mental capacities.

A study of the educational levels of persons aged 80–100 years who lived in the city of Tbilisi indicated that 44.3% were able to read and write; 14.6% had an intermediate and special education; 3.6% had a higher education; and the remainder were illiterate.

DIET

The geographic setting, along with historical tradition, greatly influence the life-styles of the longliving. One such example is in the matter of diet.

It is more through diet than any other aspect of culture that centuries-old traditions are preserved. Some of these traditions rely upon the climatic-geographic characteristics of the region.

In such a comparatively small republic as Georgia, the sharp contrast between the subtropical climate of its western zones and the continental climate of the eastern part have produced a difference in diet within the population of these two areas.

The diet of the longliving of the Caucasus is characterized by a number of distinctive features, depending on where the longliving are located. The diet differs from the coastal, to the flatlands, to the mountain regions. However, in its basic features, the diet of the longliving in almost all territories of the Caucasus shares a common feature—that of moderation. Such moderation in diet also characterizes the longliving of Azerbaijan, Dogestan, and other republics of the Caucasus, all of whom contain large numbers of the longliving (see section below regarding dietary features).

CREATIVE ACTIVITIES

Since 1948, in the House of National Creativity of Abkhazia in the city of Sukhumi, an ethnographic song-and-dance ensemble of the longliving of the republic has been in existence. There are 30 participants in the ensemble. The youngest of them, L. Kvarchelia, a singer and dancer from the village of Achandara, is 80 years old. Among the participants of the ensemble are several who are celebrated for their work. S. Katsiya, 88 years old, from the village of Adzyubzha, and G. Tarba have been proclaimed "heroes of socialist labor" for high corn (maize) yields, while 84-year-old M. Sakaniya from the village of Lykhny has been awarded the "Order of Lenin."

The national storytellers, Z. Labakhua and S. Dzheniya, have long since passed their eighth decade. M. Tarkil from the Kolkhoz Duripsh has marked his 100th year. He is retired, and often performs Abkhazian folk songs as part of the ensemble. Several years ago in Tbilisi, in the Republic Artistic Olympics, the 122-year-old Galian dancer, L. Shariya, as well as 106-year-old Ambrolaur musician D. Dzhaparidze, were prize winners.

In the village of Chabano of the Tianet region lives a 100-year-old man named Petre Gorelashvili, who has spent half his life as a shepherd. He was taught to read by other shepherds and has become an author of verse. This national storyteller expresses in his poetry the hopes and dreams of a peasant. In lyric song he tells of the modern age, brotherhood and friendship of people, the glory of work, and the bounteousness of the Georgian land.

An active participant in the artistic activity of the collective of the village of Ikalto of the Telav region of East Georgia is N. Papalashvili, who has reached the age of 98. He has several victory awards from national talent shows. He has transmitted hundreds of traditions, legends, sayings, and folk songs to the young people of the village.

The longliving who have grown wise through life experience are sought out to help in solving economic problems. In the Akhali Tskhovreba village farm of the alpine village of Zemo-Bediya of the Ochamir region, eight longliving men have been employed as economic advisors for several years. The chairman of the Kolkhoz often convenes a "soviet of elders," in which the old collective far-

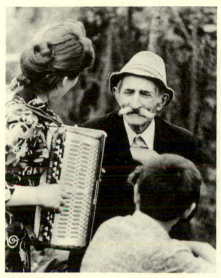 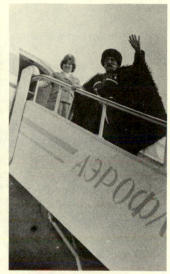

Plate 13. Georgian SSR. Samson Kachiya, 95 years old. A lover of folk songs, he is a member of the Abkhasian longliving chorus and dance ensemble "Nartaa."

Plate 14. Georgian SSR. Oldest member of the collective of the village Adzybza. 95-year-old Samson Kachiya, recipient of a special pension of merit, is pictured at the Sukhumi airport on his way to Moscow to receive the Hero of Socialist Labor award.

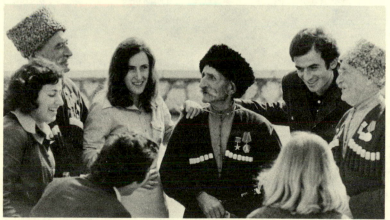

Plate 15. The longliving Samson Kachiya and a circle of friends.

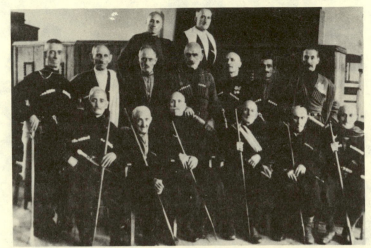

Plate 16. *Georgian SSR, Abkhasia. The longliving choral and dance ensemble, "Nartaa."*

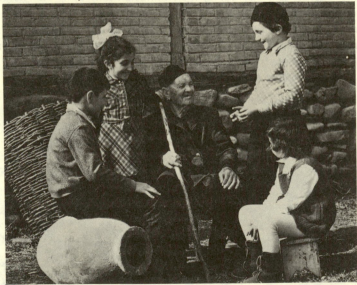

Plate 17. *S.I. Solomonishvili, the oldest collective farmer from the Vazhisubani village, recounts the history of the collective farm to some Young Pioneers. He is 102 years old.*

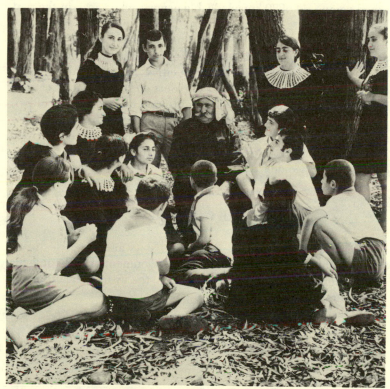

Plate 18. Georgian SSR. A veteran worker of the collective of the village Shroma in the Mazaradzhevskovo region, 80 year-old Elifan Mzaranadze is recounting the history of their native village to a group of young people.

mers discuss the problems of future developments in agriculture and provide useful counsel to the young collective farmers. At the Tasalk village workers' advisory council, a soviet of elders has been established composed of 20 knowledgable experts who were, in the past, leading producers.

On the initiative of elderly persons, many councils of retired persons have been created and are affiliated with the regional executive committees of Tbilisi and other cities, as well as the regional centers of Georgia. The councils of elders are the initiators of many benevolent activities directed at improving the well being of pensioners, along with encouraging pensioners to continue to work as long as possible. The members of the soviet (council) actively strive to lower the number of idlers and parasites—that is, anyone who lives on unearned income.

DAILY ROUTINE

Extensive observations of the work habits and life-styles of the longliving of Georgia, have led to the development of a schedule that exemplifies the daily routine followed by the average healthy longliving person living in rural setting.

Daily routine	Autumn–winter months	Spring–summer months
Rising	8:00–9:00 a.m.	7:00–8:00 a.m.
Personal hygiene, make bed, clean room	8:00–9:00 a.m.	7:00–8:00 a.m.
Morning stroll through yard (orchard, garden)	9:00–10:00 a.m.	8:00–9:00 a.m.

Breakfast	9:00–10:00 a.m.	8:00–9:00 a.m.

Work with rest breaks: a) Housework (cleaning rooms, preparing food, caring for poultry and animals) b) Work on Kolkhoz field, tea and tobacco plantations, care of citrus fruits and vineyards c) Hunting, fishing, etc.	10:00 a.m.–2:00 p.m. 11:00 a.m.–3:00 p.m.	9:00 a.m.–2:00 p.m. 10:00 a.m.–3:00 p.m.

Dinner	2:00–3:00 p.m.	3:00–4:00 p.m.

Nap	3:00–4:00 p.m.	4:00–5:00 p.m.

Housework, care of poultry and animals, sewing	4:00–6:00 p.m. 5:00–7:00 p.m.	

Supper	6:00–6:30 p.m.	7:00–7:30 p.m.

Leisure break: a) Playing with grandchildren and great-grandchildren b) Reading newspapers, listening to radio, watching television c) Visiting relatives, chatting with neighbors d) Playing on folk instruments, singing e) Evening stroll	6:30–9:00 p.m.	6:30–10:00 p.m.

Bedtime	9:00 p.m.	10:00 p.m.

The longliving are hospitable, friendly, and sociable. They are ready to come to the aid of their neighbors and to share in the sorrows and problems of friends.

Our data on some aspects of recreational and occupational activities of the longliving of the Caucasus confirm the positive effects of normal living conditions on life expectancy. A societal and familial milieu that reflects the traditions of many decades is of the utmost significance for the promotion of health and longevity.

A further study of the life-style, customs, and national traditions of the longliving of the Caucasus and other nationalities of the USSR may provide additional material for developing the most effective measures for preventing premature aging.

The outstanding revolutionary democrat D. I. Pisarev in his article, "School and Life" (1865, p. 10), wrote:

> "It is well known that the best of the contemporary medical practitioners . . . suppose that . . . all efforts of a reasonable person would not be directed toward mending and repairing the body much like a leaky ship full of holes, but toward developing a moderate life-style so that the body could maintain its healthful state and thus require repair as little as possible."

7

Health Status

The health status of the population is determined to a large degree by the demographic changes that have taken place in the USSR. In the Georgian SSR, the lowering of the birth rate and mortality, together with the increase in the average life expectancy has led to a change in the age composition of the population. As mentioned before, the numbers of persons aged 60 years and older has significantly increased.

Studies have shown that age results in a series of health changes, among these the tendency to contract chronic diseases, which are at times very difficult to treat. Aging significantly lowers the adaptive possibilities and the work capacity of the organism.

All of this leads to a number of medical and social problems, which underscore the need to significantly improve the therapeutic and preventive health-care services for all three aging categories: the mature, the old, and the longliving. There is the further need to develop for persons within these categories polyclinical and hospital assistance, as well as to further improve the operation of residences for the elderly and nursing homes. In order to develop and implement a scientifically based network of geriatric institutions and to plan preventive and therapeutic strategies, it is imperative to know the actual health status of the old and longliving.

Significant studies describing the state of health, morbidity, mortality, and problems of medical service to the elderly, were conducted by D. F. Chebotarev, Z. G. Revutskaya, N. N. Sachuk, L. A. Averbukh, Yu. I. Alabovskiy, N. V. Derkach, D. D. Gogokhi, and others. The Gerontology Center of Tbilisi, in collaboration with L. A. Dueli, D. Dzhorbenardze, A. Agadzhanov, and M. Eyderman, conducted a study of the health status of about 9,500 persons aged 80 years and older who live in the cities and villages of the republic, and 590 in the city of Tbilisi. Basically these are alert, contented persons who rarely complain of illness. Many had their first medical examination at the time of the study. They are active, jovial, interested in family matters; many actively participate in social life. About 58% of those examined looked their age; 26% looked younger; and 11% looked older.

The medical evaluation showed that 52% of the longliving were practically healthy with few complaints; 37.6% were "in poor health"; 5.71% were "frail"; 4.4% "ill"; and 1.7% "seriously ill."

According to the study, the incidence of particular diseases could be ranked as follows: diseases of the cardiovascular system (61.7%); diseases of the respiratory organs (5.4%); diseases of the nervous system (3.4%); diseases of the digestive organs (2.4%); and diseases of the genitourinary organs (2.1%). The following diseases were considered as cardiovascular pathological states: cardiosclerosis, heart defects, and hypertension.

A study of the frequency of cardiovascular diseases among highly aged urban residents revealed 130 cases of cardiosclerosis, and 95 cases of hypertension. Residents of rural areas were found to suffer cardiovascular diseases at the rate of 16 cases per 1,000 population, with 80 cases of hypertension.

From Table 7–1, it is apparent that the hypertension and myocardial infarction morbidity among urban residents is higher than among the rural, while the opposite is true of rheumatic diseases.

A study of the level of cardiovascular morbidity of the longliving by individual climatic regions of the republic was conducted in collaboration with L. Dueli. Findings indicated a relatively low level of such diseases among the longliving of western Georgia and a higher level among the longliving of eastern Georgia.

When one compares the frequency rate of cardiovascular diseases among the population as a whole with that of the longliving, one finds

Table 7-1.

Cardiovascular Morbidity Among Persons Aged 80 Years and Older
(Numbers per 100,000 Population in %)

Nosological forms of diseases	Rural Residents	urban Residents	Total
Hypertension	9.7	13.4	10.3
Myocardial infarction and angina pectoris	0.6	1.0	0.66
Rheumatic defects	19.0	17.6	18.7

that among the longliving, the hypertension and infarction morbidity is significantly higher. One should bear in mind, however, that the cardiovascular apparatus of the longliving, as the most active system, wears out simply through years of use, as well as by being subjected to pathological lesions. Only favorable living conditions and compensatory protective mechanisms developed by the organism allow these people to attain longevity, even in the presence of functional disorders.

The high actual number of cardiovascular cases within the general picture of the morbidity of the longliving—that is, the higher incidence of these diseases compared to the morbidity of the entire population—illustrates the need for therapeutic and preventive measures to be implemented for this age group.

Chronic bronchitis, pulmonary emphysema, and tuberculosis were counted as pathology of the respiratory organs. The proportion of men afflicted with chronic bronchitis (18.7%) and pulmonary emphysema (15.7%) is higher than that of women (10.5% and 10.7%). Morbidity of the respiratory organs among the longliving urban population is higher than that of the rural population.

As regards tubercular lesions of the lungs, they were observed in 1.2% of the men and 1.8% of the women. This is evidently "senile tuberculosis," which has a benign course and allows the person to live to advanced age.

The digestive and urogenital systems are less affected among the longliving: 3% to 4% in the general morbidity structure. These diseases more frequently affect men.

Diseases of the supportive-motor apparatus are found in 8.4% of the longliving (9.1% of the women, 7.8% of the men).

Among the longliving, cases of malignant neoplasms, bone tuberculosis, and venereal diseases are unusual.

The majority of the subjects (80%) were responsive, retained a good memory, and were emotionally stable. Loss of memory is noted chiefly with regard to current events, although the longliving have excellent memories for past events.

In the V. M. Bekhterev Psychoneurological Institute, I. V. Bokiy found, among 75 normal healthy persons aged 55–96 years, that 60 of the subjects had noticed a decline in memory, chiefly regarding current events. The memory of events in childhood and youth was distinctly preserved, including dates, names, and last names of people.

The loss of memory for recent events was considered by I. P. Pavlov to be a common phenomenon of physiological senescence. He considered this change to be the result of an age-specific reduction in the mobility of a special stimulation process in old age—an inertness which has its onset in old age (Pavlov, 1949, p. 440).

Some of the subjects experienced a progressive weakening of the memory as a result of the reduction of the tonus of the cerebral cortex and the sluggishness of its functional capabilities. In such longliving persons, traces of fresh stimulations (current events) disappeared first, and then the memory of remote events also dropped.

In a study of sensory loss, findings revealed that a large number of the rural longliving maintained good hearing and vision. About 74% of the longliving see well and do not wear glasses; 72% having retained auditory acuity. A certain percentage of the subjects who had experienced visual and auditory loss required special care by the family or in homes for the elderly and disabled. Such persons are provided with glasses and hearing aids.

In order to develop a scientific foundation for preventive and therapeutic strategies for the diseases of old age, it is necessary to study the causes of the mortality of the mature, the old, and the longliving.

The Gerontology Center at Tbilisi conducted a scientific analysis of

1,169 autopsy records on deceased persons of the older age groups according to the records of the First Municipal Hospital of Tbilisi (50–95 years and older). Of the deceased, 60.9% were males, 39.1% females. High mortality figures among both sexes were noted in the age group from 55 to 70 years. The highest percentage of males was in the 65-to-69-year age group (18.2%); among the females, in the 70-to-74-year age group (20%).

The study showed that causes of death ranked as follows: first, cardiovascular diseases (48.1%), second, malignant tumors (19.1%), third, genitourinary diseases (10.2%), fourth, diseases of the respiratory organs (6.5%), and fifth, digestive organs (5.5%).

Such data are also confirmed by the statistical data of the WHO on 29 countries, according to which, in most of the developed countries, the basic causes of death in old age were also cardiovascular diseases, and malignant tumors.

The main causes of death for women were atherosclerosis combined with hypertension, cancer, cholecystitis, and chronic nephritis. The largest percentage of deaths among women was made up by atherosclerosis in the 70-to-74-year age group (22.5%), whereas cases of death from myocardial infarction in the same age-sex group constituted only 8.6%. (Note: The number of women aged 70–74 dying for all causes was taken as 100%.)

Myocardial infarctions were rarely noted in the 75–79, 80–85, and

Table 7–2.

Distribution of Deaths by Causes (in %)

Cause of Death	Actual number of deaths	Males	Females
Diseases of the cardiovascular system	48.1	42.8	58.8
Malignant tumors	19.1	20.6	14.9
Genitourinary diseases	10.2	16.0	2.8
Diseases of the respiratory organs	6.5	6.8	5.8
Diseases of the digestive organs	5.5	5.4	5.3
Other diseases	10.6	8.4	12.4

older age groups. They were generally detected in the autopsies, testifying to the atypical course of diseases in the elderly.

The main causes of death for men of the older age groups were atherosclerosis, malignant tumors, prostate hypertrophy, peptic ulcer, and pneumonia. Among men, fatal outcomes of myocardial infarctions were noted more often than among women. Their largest number occurred in the 65-to-69-year age group (19.5%). In the older ages, their proportion is lower, and they were diagnosed postmortem. Among men also, atherosclerosis combined with hypertension predominates. The largest number of deaths from atherosclerosis was noted in the 75-to-79-year age group (27.3%).

Prostate hypertrophy causes relatively high mortality. In the 80-to-84-year age group, this disease, as a death cause, occupies a significant position (43.4%), a fact explained by the nature of the disease, which necessitates hospitalization and surgical intervention. The greatest number of persons dying from malignant tumors was noted in the 60-to-69-year age group.

The number dying from heart defects, cirrhosis of the liver, leukemia, and diabetes is insignificant, especially among persons of more advanced age and the longliving. Evidently, persons suffering from such diseases do not live to advanced age.

Diagnosis in patients of many diseases such as tuberculosis, nonspecific pneumonia, and myocardial infarction is less accurate in the older age groups because of their atypical course.

In Georgia, the presence of particular elements conducive to aging and longevity, such as a particular demographic pattern, the nature of the climate and geographic conditions, the standard of living, and the culture, all contribute to nurturing a large group of persons who have undergone extensive periods of physiological aging (i.e., the longliving).

Clinical studies of the longliving and experiments by Georgian gerontologists have led to the distinguishing of particular patterns followed by cardiovascular diseases. They have also been able to determine the leading role played by the nervous system in integrating and correlating the function of the organs and systems during the process of ontogenesis.

The physiological aging of the longliving is characterized by the absence of sharply pronounced declines in functional capabilities of the organism, maladaptation, notable disturbances in the interactions of the organs and systems, in the metabolic processes, and in the function of the regulatory mechanisms. At the same time, studies have shown that in some of the longliving, the functioning of the circulatory system is reduced, and as pointed out above, cardiovascular diseases have been found that harmonically lower the vital functions of the organism. An important subject for future research would be a study of the daily activities of the longliving in various climatic and geographic zones, making allowance for genetic conditioning, in order to determine what factors are conducive to the fostering of active long lives. Another important aspect would be to discover what compensatory mechanisms and environmental factors are responsible for the extended life-spans experienced by the longliving.

Studies performed in the Georgian SSR of the health status of aged persons, along with morbidity, have led to the conclusion that a large percentage of extremely old persons require both medical assistance and care outside the family. About one-third of the population aged 50 and older already regularly patronize outpatient clinics.

The nature of diseases suffered by elderly persons (lowered resistance, predominance of chronic or atypical forms of the disease) call for immediate intervention and require greater and more intensive study. There is a need for more and better qualified health-care personnel to deal with the special nature of their ailments, along with the need for an aggressive home-care program.

The absence of such a supportive health network has seriously affected the quality of medical care for the elderly. In spite of governmental policy favoring rapid development in such areas, actual health-care delivery contains many gaps.

According to the studies of Z. G. Revutskaya and N. V. Derkach, persons aged 50 years and older are sent for hospital treatment in 4.5% to 7% of the cases, when actually according to expert opinion, such care is required in 17.5% to 23% of the cases. At the 31st session of the General Convention of the USSR Academy of Medical Sciences, B. Petrovskiy, Minister of Health of the USSR, said:

Studies of the geriatric problem are of vital importance. A practical solution to such problems can only be described as urgent. In this country there are many mature and old persons who suffer from various diseases. The social significance of this problem and its medical aspects require our attention. Geriatric centers for rehabilitative and preventive care which incorporate proper recognition of the special nature of this population must be created (Petrovskiy, 1971).

The creation of a special geriatric network of rehabilitation centers and of training programs for specialists in the prevention and treatment of diseases of the elderly is being vigorously advocated. Such services must accommodate the differing needs of the three age categories: the mature, the old, and the longliving.

I. D. Bogatyrev recommends consideration of specialized hospitals and institutions, to be developed to meet particular needs such as length of stay required (short-term or long-term), the disease state, and the nature of services required. (Bogatyrev, 1972, p. 181)

Models for medical service should include periodic medical examinations and hospital observation of the mature, old, and longliving. Frequent examinations will allow for early disease detection and prompt intervention. This is of particular significance in treating such populations, since even in advanced disease states they rarely, if ever, request medical assistance. This fact became clear during an exhaustive study of persons aged 80 years and older throughout the Republic. Particular attention needs to be given to the further development of a network of homes for the elderly or disabled. Such homes are presently developed without regard for local needs and frequently do not meet minimal medical standards.

According to the studies of D. F. Chebotarev, about 200,000 persons presently reside in homes for the aged throughout the country. In 1975, more than 11% of the total population of the Soviet Union was 60 years of age or older. The presence of increasing numbers of persons of advanced age who require care outside the family calls for a significant increase in the number of institutions for the aged. Improvements are also needed in the quality of care provided in such settings.

Health-care personnel need to develop model plans incorporating work opportunities and leisure-time pursuits for a variety of residences for older persons, allowing for differences in age, state of health, and the remaining working capacity of those under care.

In Georgia where a large number of health resorts are already present, certain establishments could be assigned for treatment and restorative care of persons of retirement age and the elderly. The creation of special rehabilitation centers and the modernizing of some of the therapeutic-prophylactic institutions, geared toward therapy and disease prevention, such as clinics and health resorts, would also aid materially in the solution of these problems.

The Soviet government, in a display of concern for persons of retirement age, has recommended the adoption of measures to improve the financial status and living conditions of the retired. A resolution has been adopted for the construction of homes for the elderly and disabled totaling 73,000 units, as well as commercial retirement residences. Construction has begun on two 12-story buildings in the Khimok region on the bank of the canal in Moscow.

This is the first commercial development of retirement residences in the Russian federation. Such retirement homes will be erected in a number of the autonomous republics, regions, and provinces of the RSFSR, as well as by the Moscow and Leningrad municipal Departments of Social Security. Such residences will house men over the age of 60 and women over 55 who do not require medical care. The Social Security Departments will process housing applications and costs will range from 60 to 80 rubles ($100 to $133) per month.

The tenants of the retirement homes will live in one- or two-bedroom apartments. They will be provided with community support services and recreational opportunities. Opportunities to work in shops, garden plots, and so on, will be available. Free medical assistance will be provided. Hospital and specialized outpatient assistance, if necessary, will be provided within the commercial retirement homes by the health-care units of the health agencies.

At the same time, following the example of other nations, special retirement villages need to be organized. An example of such a town is the "old people's city," De Gamles By, located in the very center of

Copenhagen, Denmark. The town is designed for 1,560 persons. It has given shelter to old people who are capable of leading a more or less active life.

In Japan, near Tokyo, at the Atami Health Resort, celebrated for its therapeutic hot springs, a small specially designed town for 900 elderly persons has been developed.

In Vienna, in the construction by the municipalities of new residences, special blocks were selected to house older persons. In each municipality, up to 20% of the apartments are specially equipped for the elderly. In the Steinitz-Hoff region of Vienna, for example, there are about 300 apartments inhabited by old people.

8

Work:

The Source of Long Life

*I*t has naively been believed that the main factor in the preservation of health and prolongation of life is rest, or inactivity. Scientific research, however, has demonstrated that no inactive person has ever lived to an advanced age. Work serves to build health and, as such, is a decisive factor in determining long life. Laziness, idleness, and parasitism are the enemies of health and longevity.

As early as the first century of our era, the well-known Roman encyclopedist and physician Aulus Cornelius Celsus, in his work *On Medicine*, wrote: "Idleness weakens the body and work strengthens it: the first causes premature aging, the second promotes prolonged youth" (1959, p. 27).

I. R. Tarkhnishvili considered labor to be an indispensable condition of longevity. However, he asserted, most of the longliving are to be found among those who till the soil; but never among the factory workers of Russia.

"Labor," writes K. I. Parkhon, "played a decisive role in longevity. Labor created man. Labor contributed and still contributes to longevity" (1960, p. 17).

Labor enables one to preserve intellectual and physical strength, health, energy, clarity of thought, and interest in life for many years. Of the five secrets of longevity held by the longliving Azerbaijanian, Makhmud Ayvazov, the main secret of longevity was labor—the daily involvement in work.

Shirali Muslimov, a collective farmer of the Lerik region of Azerbaijan, herded sheep all his life and remained in the mountains for 15–16 hours every day. In Kabardino-Balkaria resides Chokka Zalikhanov, who is 112 years old at this writing. He has climed Mt. Elbrus 207 times.

The oldest female resident of the mountain village of Kyunkishlak in Azerbaijan, Beyim Mekhraliyeva, is 138 years old. She has engaged in physical work all of her life and now, in the autumn of her life, she helps her fellow villagers by caring for the children of peasants who are working in the fields.

Under the leadership of the Institute for Gerontology of the USSR Academy of Medical Sciences, medical examinations of more than 40,000 people aged 80 years and older have been conducted in a number of Soviet republics. According to the data obtained, all of the subjects had worked in the past and about 60% were still working at the time of the examination.

A study of the occupational history of the longliving people of Georgia shows that all of them worked in the past; about 45% of them worked for more than 50 years. More than 60% of the persons aged 80 years and older are still working according to their capacities: they work on collective farms, state farms or on citrus and tea plantations; they care for the livestock and poultry; or they participate in hunting. As a rule, all of them began working while still very young.

D. F. Chebotarev stated at the Ninth International Congress of Gerontology in Kiev that human physical and intellectual potential can be preserved only under conditions of work—that is, physical activity. The period of the "third age" should not merely have survival as its goal, but socially meaningful survival.

The staff of the Tbilisi Gerontology Center on a visit to the settlement of Digomi interviewed the collective farmer I. G. Kanadashvili. He is about 100 years old, and a kind-hearted and friendly old man. He was interviewed in his orchard, while trenching trees. In describing himself, he said:

I have a large family—a wife, 6 children, 20 grandchildren, and 40 great-grandchildren. I have been working for more than 80 years now. I love work in the same way that I love the air of our mountains and valleys. I work at the mill or as a shepherd. When they ask me what is the "secret" of long life, I answer, "work!" Laziness is the worm that undermines life!

The living conditions in the rural areas require persons to work longer than they do in the city. Work could possibly be regarded as having a beneficial effect upon rural inhabitants, for 85% of the inhabitants of rural areas are numbered among the longliving, while only 15% of the city residents figure among the number of persons throughout the republic reaching 100 years and more.

A study of participation in the work force and the functional state of the cardiovascular system of the longliving has shown that with declining work activity, a significant deterioration is noted in the functional state of the cardiovascular system. The degree of pathological damage to the cardiovascular system is directly dependent on the age and work activities of the subject.

A long history of work involvement that does not diminish with age, increases the adaptive possibilities of the hemodynamics and respiration of the body. The longliving are extremely active; many of them do extensive walking. Not one of them is overweight.

The work capacity and energy of R. R. Inaneshvili, the 112-year-old collective farmer of the village of Opshkviti of the Tskhaltub region, is incredible. He had been allotted a 2-hectare plot. Through his persistent efforts this collective farmer had attained a high yield of corn and also obtained 2.5 tons of grain. By applying an additional 2 tons of phosphorus and 10 tons of organic fertilizer to the plot, he is now about to obtain one and one-half times as much corn.

Khfaf Lasurii, from a Kolkhoz of the village Kvitouli of Ochamchir in Abkhazia, is 138 years old. She gets up with the sun as she has done for many years, rejoicing in the dawn of the working day. Even though she is well-to-do, she does not spend the day in idleness.

G. N. Kapanadze, 112 years old, lives in the settlement of Chkhirauli of the Chiatur region. Despite his age, he not only works at home, but on the Kolkhoz, stimulating the young people to a love for work. Because of his wisdom and experience, he has helped to resolve some of the economic problems of his native village.

A. G. Sulaberidze, a worker in the Gegut dairy-vegetable Sovkhoz, is more than 100 years old. He cultivates a thriving vegetable garden, and his advice is willingly received by the young vegetable gardeners of the Sovkhoz.

I. Shvangiradze, of the village of Gvishtibi of the Tskhaltub region, is 106 years old. He is mentally alert and cares for his vineyard, as well as cultivating corn. Two collective farmers of the village Etser of Samtred region—M. Kaladze, 90, and V. Kakabadze, 80—are no less active.

Epro Mikava, who is now 98 years old, works on one of the tea plantations of the village of Medani of the Tsalendzhikh region. She retired long ago, but does not plan to leave the plantation where the first tea plant was sown by her hands.

The twins Vladimir and Taras Gogoli, who have completed their 98th year, live not far from Poti. They receive a pension from the state, but continue to work on their own garden plot and look after their domestic animals.

Close to Tbilisi, in Mtskheta, M. Mamulashvili, 97 years old, works as a floriculturist. He has devoted his entire life to landscape gardening, and in his garden are found a collection of flowers that are native to many parts of the world.

Not only physical but also intellectual work promotes health and longevity. "Every hygienist," wrote A. Bebel,

> agrees to the beneficial effect of activity when balanced with mental and physical work. Only such activity is natural; it is important that it be performed in moderation and in accordance to individual ability (1959, p. 48).

Many examples can be cited to confirm that love for work, creative activity, and intellectual functioning are maintained even until advanced age. Until the very last days of their lives, many of the outstanding contributors to the worlds of science and art continued to work: Goethe, Voltaire, Hugo, Bernard Shaw, Leo Tolstoy, Edison, Mechnikov, Darwin, I. Michurin, Karpinskiy, and Dzhambul. There

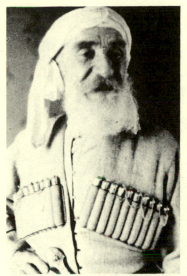 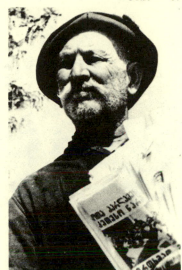

Plate 19. Georgian SSR. V. O. Kruashvili, 105 years old.
Plate 20. Georgian SSR. Mailman Serapion Paikadze, 95 years old, of the Dichashko village in the Vanskovo region.

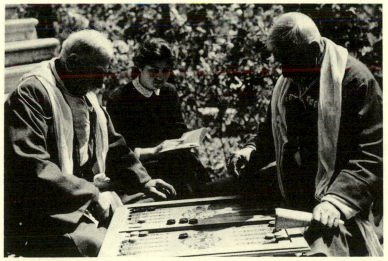

Plate 21. Georgian SSR. Twin brothers Vladimir and Taras Gogoli (city of Poti), 98 years old. Both are attractive in appearance and are physically healthy; neither one wears glasses.

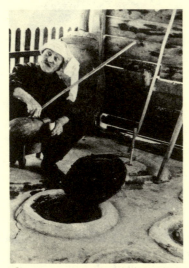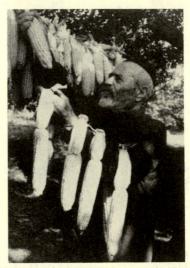

Plate 22.   Georgian SSR. E. Dolidze, an old collective farmer, in his wine cellar. He is from the Natanebi village in the Macharadzevskovo region.

Plate 23.   Georgian SSR. G. P. Tetrashvili, born in 1861, lives in the village suburb Digomi and works on the collective farm.

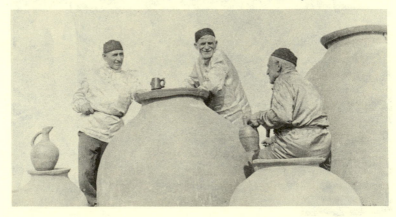

Plate 24.   Georgian SSR. Old collective farmers of the Telavskovo region at the wine cisterns.

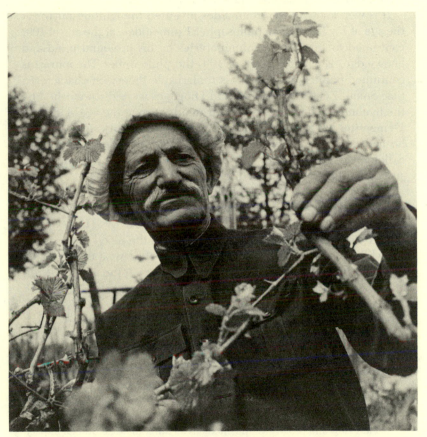

Plate 25. Georgian SSR. Old viticulturist from the collective of Alaverdi village in the Ordzonikidze Zestafonskovo region. A hero of Socialist Labor, Ilya Gachechiladze.

are many examples of outstanding works of literature and fine art that were produced at mature and even advanced ages.

It is well-known that Archimedes invented the igniting mirror at the age of 75. The Cretan philosopher Epimenides, at the age of 100, continued to amaze his contemporaries by his profound mind and knowledge. Even at the age of 100, the philosopher Theophrastus continued publicly to preach his remarkable theory on characteristics. Solon, Zeno, Pythagoras, and Diogenes were distinguished by the liveliness and freshness of their minds even at the age of 90, and Democrites never stopped ridiculing human stupidity at 95 years, as he had done even in his early youth. Plato compiled many of his dialogues at the age of 80, and Cato, upon reaching the same age, succeeded in learning the Greek language (Pineau, 1901).

Sophocles lived to the age of 90. He wrote *Oedipus Rex* at the age of 70, and *Oedipus at Colonus* at the age of 89. When Sophocles was 83 years old, he organized the defense of Athens. W. Harvey completed his magnum opus on the circulation of the blood at the age of 73, while Goethe completed the second part of *Faust* at the age of 83. Verdi lived for 88 years. He wrote *Otello* when 73, the opera *Falstaff* at age 80, and at the age of 85 the *Partitura Ge Deit*.

When L. N. Tolstoy was 82 years old, his intellect, creativity, and talent for description were fully preserved. Romains Rolland stated:

> Intellectual alertness is also evident in the stories written during the very last illness suffered by Tolstoy. Almost until the end of his life, he continued to write daily or to dictate his diary. We are struck by the intellectual force which Tolstoy preserved to his last day. In every description of human action or a personage, he remains an artist with an eagle's view and broad sweep which has an immediate emotional impact. He never loses this majestic clarity of thought. The unique example of a great artist in the full flower of creative force (n.d., p. 326).

At the age of 103, the president of the Medical Academy, Alexander Genio, died in Paris. With a perfectly clear mind, he worked intensely to the last days of his life.

The well-known Austrian psychiatrist, Nobel Prize winner Ju. Wagner-Jaureg, died at the age of 84. After his death, a manuscript was found on his desk indicating that until the end of his life he had been working on the problem of longevity.

Bernard Shaw lived almost to the age of 100, and continued to work up to the last days of his life. "The best way to be happy," he said, "is to work intensely, to try to be of use to people." The physiologist Charles Sherrington lived to the age of 93 and worked all of his life.

The well-known Russian microbiologist S. N. Vinogradskiy died at the age of 97. During the last days of his life, he was proofreading his new book. The writer and scholar N. A. Rubakin died at the age of 84 and until his last day was writing a new book on educational psychology. Throughout his last years, according to his son, Professor A. N. Rubakin, he worked from 6 A.M. until evening, as he had done much of his life.

I. P. Pavlov completed his works, *Twenty years of experience in the objective study of the higher nervous activity (behavior) of animals, Conditioned reflexes,* and *Lectures on the work of the cerebral hemispheres* between the ages of 74 and 78.

The former dean of Canterbury Cathedral, the well-known English progressive and recipient of the Lenin Prize "For strengthening peace between peoples," Hulett Johnson, died at the age of 92. Even in the last days of his life, he was a vigorous advocate of peace and participated actively in the world peace council.

The hygienist-gerontologist academician Z. G. Frenkel of the USSR Academy of Medical Sciences retained his intellectual capacity almost until his death at the age of 100. During the last period of his life, his schedule was as follows:

> Get up at 5:30, calisthenics, bodymassage, then "latest news" on the radio. At 9:30, breakfast and a stroll. At 12, secretary arrives and work begins until 4 o'clock: They read to me and I dictate. After dinner, a small rest and meetings with visitors, students, and friends. At 8 p.m., supper, radio, telephone conversations with relatives. At 11:30, go to bed

In 1956, a study was made of the activities of a number of well-known scholars in different branches of science. The group examined included 17 astronomers, 24 chemists, 19 geologists, 17 mathematicians, 34 biologists, 17 physicians, 20 physicists, and 10 scholars in other sciences, totaling 158 men.

At the age of 20 to 29 years, each of them had individually published an average of nine scientific works. Ninety-six of the scientists had begun to publish only at the age of 25 and older. Between the ages of 30 and 39 years, they wrote an average of 20 articles per year, and in the next 20 years from 20 to 24 articles. Between the ages of 60 and 70, the number of articles published by them dropped to 18, and at the age of 80 years and above, to 13 articles per year. Thus, even after 80 years, the publications of these scientists was greater than when aged 30 or under (Rubakin, 1966, pp. 138–139).

In February 1971, a sketch was broadcast on the All-Union Radio that had been prepared by the literary editorial staff of Georgian radio concerning the 98-year-old student Nike Papalashvili, who had recently completed the 2-year course of the Ikaltoy People's University of Culture. The list of intellectually active persons who continued creative work at an advanced age is long.

Even Ch. Hufeland when describing the longevity of persons engaged primarily in intellectual pursuits, remarked that among physicians, mortality is high and that they, by the nature of their occupation, cannot live long.

It is unjust that it should be physicians, for it is they who provide others with the opportunities for the preservation of life and health. But unfortunately, in fact, it is not so. The proverb "serving others they become exhausted, benefiting others, they die" . . . seems to refer to physicians. (Hufeland, 1853, p. 178)

With respect to mortality and the life expectancy of persons of various occupations, I. R. Tarkhnishvili also asserted that

physicians experience a very high mortality, and this is, of course, understandable if we take into account the life-style of the majority of doctors who are continually exposed to infectious diseases and who are obliged to respond, day and night, to suffering. Physicians are further constantly concerned with the fate of persons who have entrusted their lives to them.

Concerning longevity among doctors, I. R. Tarkhnishvili lists the names of doctors who have lived to 100 years and more. He writes that despite the high mortality and short life expectancy of doctors, "nevertheless one encounters many fortunate ones who, thanks to the laws of heredity or to good health care and a positive attitude, do reach advanced age" (Tarkhnishvili, 1903).

Studies have shown that any work—whether intellectual or physical—if it provides personal satisfaction and supports the public good, contributes to continued good health and long life. From this it follows that a person who wishes to live long should be engaged in socially useful work until old age. I. V. Davydovskiy wrote:

> We should build into the consciousness of people the conviction expressed repeatedly by ancient writers and philosophers that work is not only happiness, but health; work is a form of prevention against "premature aging" (1966, p. 10).

In order to preserve the capacity to work, to build health, and to attain a long life, one must maintain the correct diet, a balanced daily routine, and a regular schedule of work and rest; all contribute to the effective regulation of the total organism. Scientific studies indicate that any disturbance in the balance of work and rest through emergencies or overwork is damaging to health. Proper intervals of rest eliminate fatigue and protect the body against wear and tear.

Health and long life are promoted not only by physical work, but by intellectual work as well. Intense cerebral activity for many years, while still observing the rules of health, does not exhaust the nervous system, but rather strengthens it. The notion that the intellectual efforts of engineers, doctors, teachers, and creative persons such as writers, artists, and composers depend solely upon talent and inspiration is erroneous. Only through organization and planning and a reasonable distribution of working time can one become maximally productive, and yet maintain good health over a long period of time.

Outstanding scientists, literary figures, artists, and politicians have always valued their time. According to a life-style developed over many years, they devoted time not only to recreation, but also to intensive work without causing damage to their health and without reducing the pace of their activities.

Failure to consider the physical requirements connected with intensive work leads to chronic overfatigue. Such a negligent attitude toward the nervous system undermines health and accelerates the onset of aging. As a result, susceptibility to disease is much higher, leading to a concomitant drop in working capacity.

Scientists at the Institute of Gerontology of the USSR Academy of Medical Sciences, in studying the health status of about 500 scientists in Moscow aged 60–75 years, found that the majority of the subjects did not observe an orderly schedule of work and rest. They overburdened themselves with work by holding down two jobs and working on their days off and during vacation. It is not surprising, as D. F. Chebotarev writes, that many post-middle-aged scientists have suffered from diseases of the cardiovascular system, primarily atherosclerosis.

The Russian physiologist, N. Ye. Vvedenskiy, has developed a set of five conditions for increasing mental working capacity:

1. A gradual assumption of the task
2. Moderation and the development of a rhythm suited to the task
3. Development of an orderly and systematic approach
4. Alternating periods of work and rest with changes of work focus
5. A favorable public disposition toward the work in progress.

"Every time you begin a complicated job," writes I. P. Pavlov, "never hurry, take your time, evaluate the task, develop a sensible schedule to avoid frustration."

Work that is improperly organized can bring on fatigue—that is, a physiological state that, as I. M. Sechenov demonstrated, results from a disturbance in the activity of the nerve cells of the cerebral cortex. The first signs of fatigue initiate the process of inhibition that counteracts the development of fatigue. The inhibitory process protects the nerve cell from fatigue resulting from certain functional disorganizations. Fatigue is a temporary disturbance of bodily functions, while inhibition is an indispensable physiological process necessary to the operation of our nervous system. The processes of arousal are clearly manifest when a person is awake, while the processes of inhibition occur during sleep.

Controlling fatigue in order to further increase work productivity can be accomplished through the improvement of working conditions. Cleanliness and order, proper ventilation and illumination in the work areas, and elimination of noise and vibration, are all factors that reflect positively upon the human organism, particularly of those who are past middle-age. The development of a work rhythm that balances the expenditure and conservation of effort is of great importance as well.

Exercise and physical conditioning play a significant role in the control of fatigue. I. P. Pavlov, in his remarkable theory, "On the Dynamic Sterotype," (1949, v. 1, p. 142) showed how exercise promotes fatigue control. I. P. Pavlov defined as a sterotype the system of conditional reflexes that are expressed through any action, such as working on an assembly line, washing, eating, and so on. Numerous studies have shown that retirement—the cessation of work activity—brings about a disturbance of the accustomed pattern and rhythm of life, thus changing the dynamic stereotype. This leads to a progressive reduction in the potential for development of the organism that is then reflected in a number of physiological ways. A change in the life-style established over the course of years, such as the cessation of work activity, leads to a rapid onset of senescence. For old persons, the transition to lighter work is much more difficult than would be continuing the same work, even if the nature of the task is more complex.

Numerous studies performed on different groups of muscles have shown that in old age, muscular strength declines noticeably, and at the age of 50 years, it amounts to 30% of the strength of the muscles of a 20-year-old youth. After 60 years, the circulatory efficiency declines in the muscles, chiefly in the myocardium, and the muscle tonus at rest declines much more rapidly.

New sterotypes are developed easily and rapidly in the young and healthy who possess strong nervous systems. In the middle-aged and ill, however, if the established sterotypes are extremely stable, new sterotypes are developed with difficulty. "Any office worker," said I.

P. Pavlov, citing an example, "works at his simple job without problems until 70, but once he retires and disturbs the life sterotype, his body stops functioning regularly, and he soon dies" (Pavlov, 1949, p. 142).

A. Serenko and G. Tsaregorodtsev emphasize that with increasing age, it is more difficult for a person to alter the established dynamic sterotype. This means, in effect, that changing occupational roles and orientation in old age must correspond to former work roles to avoid discontinuity. Such correspondence must take into account physical states and age changes. Systematic exercise and training can assist post-middle-aged persons to develop a dynamic sterotype—that is, a set of operations reinforced by conditional reflex ties.

The above data indicate that the preservation of work capabilities in the periods of maturity, old age, and the longliving can be effected when certain factors are given proper consideration. Such factors include a healthy life-style combined with favorable external environmental conditions. These conditions are indispensable for the preservation of health and the prolongation of life.

9
Diet

Not only work, but proper nutrition, diet, and meal scheduling have great importance for health and long life. It is well known that in maturity and old age, the metabolic processes decline, the body weight decreases, motor activity and the self-restorative processes of the body are reduced, and concomitant diseases often appear. Therefore, a properly balanced diet, comprising the basic food components, will aid in the preservation of health and prevent premature aging.

In collaboration with D. Dzhorbenadze, M. Aurabashvilli, and A. Agadzhanov, the Tbilisi Gerontology Center investigated the dietary habits of the old and longliving in the regions of eastern and western Georgia. This was the first attempt to study the actual diet of the old and longliving within two different climatic-geographic zones of the republic of Soviet Georgia.

A study of nutrition among the longliving resulted in the finding that a mixed diet is found in 85% of the population, a lactovegetarian diet in 8% to 10%, and a meat diet in only 5% to 7%. Their diet is, by and large, of a moderate nature. The caloric content of the diet was somewhat lower than that recommended for this age group, which may in part explain the absence of overweight persons among them. During the past decades, the longliving have not exhibited any sharp fluctations in weight, a fact further corroborated by their moderate diet and high level of physical activity.

The average daily diet of the subjects consisted predominantly of vegetables. This was truer of the eastern regions of the republic. The diet contained a large portion of raw vegetables eaten in the form of salads. They also eat a variety of fresh greens, rich in vitamins and minerals, such as cress, coriander, tarragon, dill, green onions, fennel, garlic, and so on. Besides vegetables, the longliving consume quantities of fruit, citrus fruits, and dried sweet herbs. The latter are used in large quantities throughout the year, saturating the diet with vitamin C, which is of particular importance in old age. Such a diet might also partially explain the relatively low proportion of persons suffering from atherosclerosis and its mild course, when found, among the longliving.

In Georgia along with cultivated varieties of vegetables, dishes are prepared from wild edible plants that are rich in vitamins and mineral salts. These vegetable dishes have good enzyme attackability, which has a beneficial effect upon the reduced functional capabilities of the digestive system in old age.

The longliving of Nagornyy Karabakh of the Azerbaijan SSR are accustomed to eating many wild edible plants in a variety of forms: cooked, pickled, or raw. These plants are very rich in vitamins of the B group, nicotinic and ascorbic acids, and vitamin E. Ripe shakhtut berries are also a prominent feature in their diets. These berries, which contain, besides vitamin C, up to 30% sugar, are regarded as very beneficial in cardiovascular diseases. In the mountain villages, it is customary to brew tea from the berries of the briar and the flowers of the hawthorne, linden, and strawberry.

In western Georgia, all kinds of broths rich in extractive substances undesirable in old age, are avoided. Meat such as boiled chicken and beef, and on occasion mutton, is generally eaten. Boiling meat is more suitable than other methods of preparation for the digestion, in view of the reduction of the enzyme activity of the glands of the alimentary tract in old age.

In the coastal regions of western Georgia, a large part of the diet is composed of plant and fish products, as well as chicken. In the mountain regions, a milk–meat diet predominates. In place of white bread, cornmeal and hominy are preferred.

The longliving of the mountain regions of Azerbaijan-Nagornyy Karabakh and the Nakhichevian ASSR—in contrast to the longliving of Georgia—eat beef and chicken, but prefer mutton. Despite this, the cholesterol level in the blood of this group of the longliving is not high.

Although the longliving of western and eastern Georgia consume predominantly boiled meat, the longliving of Azerbaijan do not give up their traditional shashlik. The animal protein requirement is basically satisfied by milk and dairy products. The favorite food of the Azerbaijan longliving is fermented milk with garlic, and also as a first-course, skim whey rich in protein and mineral salts. The regular consumption of products containing lipotropic substances—milk, sour milk (matsoni), cheese, as well as vegetables and fruits—creates the antisclerotic basis of the diet of the persons studied.

A good source of animal protein is the cheese that the longliving consume in large quantities. Cheese contains protective amino acids, which are of vital necessity in old age; as well as calcium, which is important in the prevention of senile osteoporosis. In the daily diet of the longliving, sour milk (matsoni) is found in large quantities, whereas the consumption of milk is relatively low.

A certain contradiction appears with respect to gerodietetics in terms of the consumption by the old people of the eastern regions of Georgia of relatively high quantities of animal fats. The consumption of melted tallow is a characteristic feature of the diet of the population of the eastern regions of the republic. However, the actual amount of vegetable fats used in western Georgia is greater than the animal fats. The population of this area uses large quantities of a local variety of Greek walnut, which contains 51.9% to 69.9% fat, as a shortening.

The normal diet of the longliving can be regarded as consisting of natural products of their own preparation (cheese, sour milk, hominy, cornmeal, bread, etc.). The products are cooked fresh without being subjected to refrigeration. The hot dishes are consumed immediately after preparation, preventing the destruction of vitamins that occurs during the storage and reheating of food. According to national custom and tradition, the longliving use spicy seasonings of red and black pepper in the form of sauces—such as wild plum sauce (tkemali), walnut sauce (bazhi), a pungent paste of walnuts, red pepper and various condiments (ajika)—which stimulate the appetite and improve the flavor of dishes.

The longliving of Georgia consume little sugar (which has little dietary significance and produces only a certain number of calories and energy), instead they consume quantities of natural honey, which is rich in vitamins and is a protection against many diseases and an important factor in longevity. They also eat large quantities of grapes.

Following a centuries-old tradition, in contrast to the longliving of other nationalities of the Causasus, the longliving of Georgia always drink a moderate amount of home-made wine before meals.

In the mountain settlements of Azerbaijan, Dagestan, and southern Ossetia, as well as that part of Georgia (Adzharia and partially Abkhazia), where the population practiced the Moslem religion in the past, the longliving never consume alcoholic beverages. Pure mountain spring water, in the words of the longliving of these republics, is good for the digestion, provides energy and alertness, and promotes long life.

The longliving of Georgia, in the majority, have not smoked and do not smoke. The smokers usually stop smoking by the age of 50–70, because they are aware of the harmful effects of nicotine upon health.

The eating habits of the old merit attention. As a rule, they eat three to four times a day at specific times, and they never eat to satiety. They believe that "it is better to undereat than overeat." The greatest amount of food is consumed at mid-day.

The absence of metabolic disturbances in the individuals studied, as well as their high motor activity, testify to the relatively well-balanced nature of the basic food components of their diet. Studies indicate that the diet of the rural population of the old and longliving of western Georgia, on the whole, corresponds better to contemporary dietary recommendations than the diet of the same age groups of the eastern regions of the republic. The greater life expectancy in the western regions of Georgia can be explained to a certain degree by their dietary rules, which play a significant role in the complex of factors that influence human life expectancy.

At the present moment it is difficult to ascertain whether the ideal

diet promotes more rapid growth, or a longer life span, or a prolonged period of absence of disease, or the greatest ability to adapt to
unfavorable environmental conditions. At any rate, the dietary factor, seen in its proper role along with other external environmental
factors, conditions not only the health and life expectancy, but also
the length of productive human life.

In order to maintain health and working capacity in old age—to
achieve long life—a properly balanced diet is of the utmost importance. Diet must conform to the alterations in the physiological and
biochemical systems of the body and maintain their functioning at full
capacity. In order to prevent premature aging, a proper diet should
be initiated by approximately the age of 45–50 years, when one
begins, more or less, to notice the first "precursors" of physical aging.
It is no secret that a scientifically well-balanced diet is capable of
preventing the development of atherosclerosis and its complications,
metabolic diseases, especially obesity and digestive disturbances—
which are frequent companions of the second half of human life.

But how should one eat in old age in order to remain hale and
hearty?

Unhealthful and harmful dietary habits and tastes should be
changed gradually. Foods damaging to the mature and old should be
replaced by beneficial ones, even if they were not customarily consumed in earlier years. A standard rule for the mature and old should
be moderation in eating. The necessity of reducing the caloric intake
with age is due to the reduction of physical mobility and in muscular
weight of the body, as well as the decline of the metabolic processes
in old age.

Getting fat is harmful to the health! Excessive weight is an un-
necessary load on the organism, its heart and blood vessels. At the
same time, excess weight, is in the majority of cases, accompanied by
an increase in the production of cholesterol by the body, thus promoting the development of early atherosclerosis. Only by observing
moderation in eating at this age can one prevent an increase in
weight, which is extremely harmful to health. Obesity and overeating in the mature and old lead to serious diseases: atherosclerosis,
diabetes, gout, cholecystitis, and so on. Obesity has been condemn-
ed for many centuries. In ancient Rome, on a monument over

the grave of a man who died at the age of 112 is the laconic phrase: "He ate and drank in moderation."

In cases of obesity, the heart is poorly supplied with blood from the greatly branched vascular system that results from the tremendous size of the overweight body. Overweight persons move little, resulting in poor conditioning of the heart muscle and body muscles. They suffer from dyspnea, that is, they breathe poorly because fat impedes the movement of the diaphragm. Therefore, the control of overweight by sensible diet and physical exercise is among the primary preventive measures to be observed.

One of the celebrated representatives of the Salerno school of medicine, Arnold of Villanova (1235–1311), in his poem *Regimen Sanitatis Salernitanum*, wrote:

If you wish health to return,
And not to know disease,
Drive away the weight of care,
And consider anger to be unworthy;
Eat modestly, eschewing wine,
Do not consider valueless
Wakefulness after dining,
Scorning the afternoon nap;
Do not retain your urine long,
Nor strain at stool;
If you will follow this—you will live long in the world.
If there are too few physicians, let your physicians be
Three: Cheerful nature, tranquility, and moderate diet (1970).

The other extreme—undereating—is also harmful. I. P. Pavlov ascribed great importance to proper food and diet: "If an excessive and exclusive attraction to food is animalism, then a high degree of inattention to food is stupidity, but the truth here, as always, lies in the middle: Do not be carried away, but pay due attention" (Pavlov, 1951, p. 100).

If the calorie content of food ingested at age 30 is taken as 100%, then by the age of 70, it is advisable to reduce it to 70%, by eliminating principally animal fats and carbohydrates. One should never reduce the quantity of protein in the diet, since the aging organism suffers significant decline in the synthesis of tissues, the structural material of which is protein. One gram of protein per one kilogram body weight is the optimal protein standard for persons over 70. Proteins of skim milk, sour milk (matsoni), cottage cheese, and cheese are of particular value, since they contain substances that prevent the development of atherosclerosis.

It is well known that, due to the reduced secretion of the digestive glands in old age, putrefactive microflora begin to accumulate in the intestine, leading to an increased production of putrefactive products and their absorption into the blood. Therefore, sour milk products (matsoni, kefir [fermented milk], etc.), which suppress the activity of microbes, are highly recommended in large quantities in the diets of persons of mature and old age. The products of lactic acid fermentation (fermented milk, curdled milk, acidophylus) restore the microflora that is naturally found in younger ages to the intestine of the mature person, and harmonize intestinal function.

Milk is a valuable nutritional product. I. P. Pavlov believed that milk is the "the lightest food." A distinctive and very valuable property of milk is its easy digestability. It contains high-quality protein, a significant quantity of fats, mineral salts important for the vital activities of the body, trace elements, and vitamins.

Milk contains A, E, and B-group vitamins, as well as choline and methionine, which play a certain role in the prevention and treatment of atherosclerosis. Hypercholesterolemia is reduced as a result of milk's lecithin content. A liter of milk provides the daily requirement of animal protein for an adult who does not engage in heavy physical work, and covers about 30% of the physiological standard for fat. These qualities permit the inclusion of milk in restricted diets for persons of mature age and in special diets that are recommended for the treatment of atherosclerosis, hypertension, and diseases of the liver and gallbladder (Marshak, 1959, p. 25).

Meat should be consumed moderately, but not excluded from the diet. Immoderate consumption of meat leads to the risk of depositing salts in the joints. Protein from fish—especially ocean fish—is very useful because of the significant quantity of iodine, which has a therapeutic-preventive effect in atherosclerosis. Meat and fish are best eaten in boiled form. Also one should not totally eliminate egg protein from the diet of the elderly, as it is easily assimilated by the tissues. It has been proven that the quantity of cholesterol ingested together with egg yolk is many times less than the quantity synthesized by the body itself. Therefore, the eating of eggs no more than two to three times a week represents no particular danger with respect to the development of atherosclerosis.

In the mature age groups, the intake of fats should be limited. Fats should be consumed in a quantity of one gram fat per kilogram of body weight—that is, no more than 70–80 gm per day, including the quantity used in the preparation of food. The most appropriate ratio is 70% animal and 30% vegetable fats.

Corn and sunflower oils, which possess an antisclerotic effect, are especially useful; they do not contain cholesterol that can be deposited in the walls of the blood vessels and thus cause atherosclerosis.

To prevent obesity, one should also limit the intake of the carbohydrates, which are especially easily assimilable, such as sugar, candies, and so forth. For older persons, the total quantity of carbohydrates should not exceed 280–320 gm per day. At the same time, fructose—the sugar of fruits and berries—should be consumed in considerable quantities. The recommended standard for sugar is no more than 35 gm per day.

Sugar in larger quantities is harmful. Instead of sugar, honey, raisins, and dates (which contain natural sugars) should be recommended. Only dates can compete with honey in caloric content. The daily consumption of natural honey should become a rule for the mature person.

Vegetables, fruits, and berries are an especially valuable component in the diet of persons of the older age groups. Their cellulose content promotes the highest degree of normalization of the intestinal microflora, (as well as intestinal motor function), thus preventing constipation. A sufficient quantity of raw vegetables, fruits, and berries provides the elderly organism with vitamin C, which prevents atherosclerosis. Especially rich in vitamin C among the fruits are rose hips, black currants, citrus fruits, and apples (especially tart winter apples); of the vegetables—tomatoes, green onions, red pepper, potatoes, cabbage, and so on. Prepared vitamins are advisable when indicated by a physician. The organism of the aged person reacts sharply to disturbances in the water-salt metabolism; therefore, it requires about 2 liters of water per day, including the water contained in food. Only in cases of pronounced edema and obesity should the quantity of water be limited. The consumption of salt must be reduced to 3–4 gm per day.

Pure grape wine is recommended for elderly persons in extremely moderate quantities. This does not disturb the body functions, but raises its general tonus and promotes health. The abuse of alcoholic beverages and tobacco has a very harmful effect on the entire body and its nervous system.

It is most advisable for the old person to eat four times per day, and just as important that meals be eaten at the same time every day. In the case of a four-meal schedule, the first breakfast should contain 25% of the entire daily allowance, the second breakfast about 15%, lunch about 40%, and dinner 20%. It is harmful to begin the working day on an empty stomach, as this has a negative effect on working capacity. Persons inclined to obesity should eat five to six times per day in small portions.

It should be emphasized that a proper diet is not only moderate, but also varied and regular. A diet organized in this fashion helps retard the aging process and prevents a number of metabolic diseases.

10

Heredity and Longevity

The science of heredity began to develop at the beginning of this century. Studies by many investigators, as well as experiments in decoding the phenomena of heredity on the molecular level, have shown that the primary information on the development of hereditary characteristics is contained in the chromosomes, which are incorporated in the nuclei of the cells.

The specific component of the hereditary material of the chromosomes is deoxyribonucleic acid (DNA), which controls, through the mediation of ribonucleic acid (RNA), the primary processes of protein synthesis in the cell. It has been shown that the hereditary material of the chromosomes or genes and the primary hereditary structure of the gene consist of a group of nucleotides—that is, a gene is a small segment of a DNA molecule.

Hereditary change is simply a change in one nucleotide or a change in the order of positioning of the nucleotides in the DNA molecule. S. Alikhanyan writes of contemporary genetics:

Defining genes as the element of hereditary structure . . . does not eliminate the role of the external environment in the formation of the organism. On the contrary, it confirms that the properties of organisms are conditioned not only by their genetic constitution, but also by the environment, i.e., by various external conditions to which the organism is exposed during its development. Consequently, one does not inherit particular characteristics but standard reactions to different external conditions.

A number of investigators, on the basis of an analysis of family trees, have found that a regular relationship exists between the life expectancy of the parents and that of their offspring. L. Binet and F. Bourlier cite the data of Birren, Pearson, and Pearl, who called attention to the fact that longevity is inherited. In the classic work by Pearl, men who lived to the age of 90–100 years had had longliving ancestors. L. Binet and F. Bourlier believe that "the role of heredity in determining the maximum human life expectancy is quite evident." (Binet and Bourlier, 1960, p. 34)

Roessl, Henschel and Boening, in studying the family trees of the gynecologist Schultze and the natural scientist Heckel also found many instances of survival to advanced age, as well as a high fertility rate in longliving families. (Nagornyy, Nikitin and Bulankin, 1963, pp. 642, 644)

Other scientists, who consider the role of heredity as clearly determining the maximum human life expectancy envision a different role for each of the parents in the transmission of the tendency toward longevity to offspring. Pearl believed that "a small subgroup of exceptionally longlived subjects in a given population is biologically distinguished from the remaining mass of the population," and cited examples proving that marriages between the longliving also produce more longliving offspring. For example, in analyzing family trees of American married couples, 86% of those who have lived to the age of 90 or 100 had had one or two longlived parents (V. Nikitin).

E. Jalavista asserts that in each of the parents, the tendency to transmit longevity differs. Studying the pedigrees of prosperous Swedish and Finnish families, particularly the life expectancy of their ancestors on the paternal and maternal sides, the author found that the average life expectancy of the children is directly proportional to the life expectancy of the mother. The relationship of life expectancy in children, especially girls, to the life expectancy of the father, is less clearly indicated.

D. Niel and V. Shell write:

The problem of the degree of possible effects of environmental factors on the manifestation of the genotype represents one of the oldest problems of biology. Unfortunately, in the past when this problem was discussed, there appeared more tendentiousness than perspicacity. . . . This tendency has not been so clearly revealed in any other field than the discussion of the problem of the relative role of heredity and environment. (Niel and Shell, 1961, p. 1010)

Niel and Shell believe that although research can be performed on animals to clarify the role of environment and heredity,

Society does not permit the carrying out of strictly controlled experiments on the effect of environmental changes on human growth and development. Therefore, when studying human populations, it is practically impossible to create conditions which would permit any degree of accuracy in determining the relative role of heredity and environment in human physiology and pathology.

I. R. Tarkhnishvili believed that the length of human life depends not only on heredity, constitutional factors, and physiological functions, but also on external environmental factors. Tarkhnishvili thus sees the entire organism, including the complex biological processes taking place within it, as continuously reacting to the external environment. Emphasizing the duality of environmental factors—internal (defined by hereditary characteristics) and external (the environment in which the organism lives)—I. R. Tarkhnishvili correctly maintained that the combination of both internal and external factors determined life expectancy.

Z. G. Frenkel (1949) writes that longevity of persons with long-lived parents cannot be attributed to heredity as Pearl and Dublin had stated.

The fact that both parents in a certain group of families have lived to advanced age in itself testifies not so much to hereditary longevity as to the fact that these families lived under more favorable conditions such as the absence of exposure to fatal illnesses, the provision of better health care, and enjoyed a higher standard of living (diet, housing, sobriety, etc.).

In the opinion of A. Nagornyy, life expectancy is the result of a complicated interweaving of two distinct factors: endogenous (defined by the hereditary structure of the organism) and exogenous (determined by the properties of "that environment in which the organism lives"). The role of the hereditary factor is further complicated by the presence in higher organisms of nervous and endocrine systems. At the same time, Nogornyy concludes that existing studies indicate rather convincingly that life expectancy can be both increased and decreased by external factors. (Nagorny, 1950, p. 38) This idea is confirmed by L. Binet and F. Bourlier, who believe that "if heredity determines the potential life expectancy of the individual to a significant degree, then numerous environmental factors (ecological factors) influence the actual life expectancy."(Binet and Bourlier, 1960, p. 33)

According to the data of the Institute of Gerontology of the USSR Academy of Medical Sciences, in the Ukraine, in 40% of the persons studied, the parents were long lived; in Moldavia in 28% of the cases; and in Abkhazia in 31% (Sachuk, 1972).

R. Sh. Alikishiyev, who studied longevity among the inhabitants of Dagestan, found that in 59 out of 200 longlived persons, the parents and close relatives had also been distinguished by longevity and had survived to more than 100 years. (Alikishiyev, 1962, p. 19)

In Tbilisi, a study was made of data on hereditary longevity in 2,468 persons age 90 years and older. The hereditary factor was established in 1,184 persons (48%)—524 men and 660 women. Findings did not indicate a predominance of longevity either on the maternal or paternal side. Of 1,184 longlived persons, 948 (about 80%), although they had had longliving ancestors, were also the firstborn in their families; whereas among 1,284 longlived persons in whom the hereditary factor was not found, only 694 were the firstborn in the family (about 54%).

Table 10–1 demonstrates that longlived ancestors, including close

Table 10-1

Distribution of Longevity Among Ancestors of 1,184 Persons

No. persons of each sex	Age of parents(yrs.)	Longevity in family							
		Father	Mother	Brother	Sister	Grand-father	Grand-mother	Uncle	Aunt
Men (524)	80–89	67	63	55	36	38	53	25	7
	90+	75	46	56	43	67	59	19	16
Women (660)	80–89	113	48	67	25	51	61	38	10
	90+	86	82	25	36	48	51	29	31
	Total	341	239	203	140	204	224	111	54

relatives, were found among 757 persons aged 80–89 years, and in 759 persons aged 90 years or older. Among the 1,184 persons, there were 1,516 longlived persons (715 men, 801 women) in the family.

Listed below are data on the longevity of the families of persons studied who were 80 years of age or older.

Tskhaltubo: N. Beradze, 91 years; father, 95; mother, 90; sister, 105; brother, 86. Paternal grandparents: grandmother, 105; grandfather, 95. Maternal grandparents: grandmother, 82; grandfather, 84.

Terzhola: K. Kezevadze, 91 years; father, 120; mother, 110; sister, 100; another sister, 95.

Kvareli: M. Miminoshvili, 96 years; father, 120; mother, 117; brother, 90; sister, 82.

V. Galasvili, 85 years; father, 120; mother, 120; sister, 81; another sister, 87.

Tsageri: P. Akhvlediani, 100 years; father, 95; mother, 85. Paternal granparents: grandmother, 86; grandfather, 100. Maternal grandparents: grandmother, 84; grandfather, 90.

Lagodekhi: S. Chachanidze, 90 years; father, 100; mother, 120; brother, 80. S. Gobozov, 86 years; father, 120; mother, 100.

Khashuri: D. Dzhanashvili, 85 years; father, 100; mother, 90.

Tetri Tskaro: Sh. Elibekov, 86 years; father, 90; mother, 90; brother, 93, etc.

The great number of studies conducted in this area, along with the data of the Tbilisi Gerontology Center, strongly support the conclusion that heredity plays a certain role in human life expectancy. The data also indicate that the length of human life is predetermined by exposure to exogenous factors—factors of the external environment. Socioeconomic factors play a significant role as well.

11

Sex and the Longliving

The problems of sexual potency of the longliving have not been adequately discussed in the literature. The decline in sexual function represents only one of many signs of aging.

Involution of the sexual function in men occurs more slowly than in women. The weakening of the sexual function may be extended over several years. In the majority of cases, no sudden changes comparable to the symptoms of the climacteric in women are observed in men.

The gradual loss of sexual potency in aging men is related not only to the involution of the sexual glands, but to the general decline of physical capabilities and mental activity as well. Sexual potency depends concomitantly upon the condition of the organism as a whole, and in particular, on the glands of internal secretion that regulate sexual function. The neuroendocrine regulation of the sexual system in old age undergoes certain age-specific changes. These changes involve the pituitary, the gland that stimulates and coordinates the function of the other glands; this in turn influences the processes of growth and reproduction, carbohydrate, fat, and protein metabolism, and a number of other functions of the body. One of the important functions of the pituitary is the production of gonadotropic hormones, which are the basic stimulators of the activity of the sexual glands and of the entire sexual system (M. Yules, I. Khollo, pp. 313, 316).

F. Bourlier believes that the reduction of sexual activity among the elderly is related to various, not only endocrine, but psychological and social factors, as well. (Binet and Bourlier, pp. 375, 376)

Sometimes, however, even in greatly advanced age, there may be an unexpected restoration of sexual activity, but this is usually temporary and lasts only a few months. In extremely old men, the sperm preserves its fertilizing force, and even many years after cessation of the sex life, one can find normal spermatozoans in the semen, a fact confirmed by spermatograms.

Many investigators have noted that in the longliving, sexual activity is limited as a rule; but also, that sexual potency is preserved for a long time. (Ch. Hufeland, 1853, p. 251). I. R. Tarkhnishvili wrote: "All people who have lived to reach advanced ages retain a high reproductive capacity, and at times this capacity continues until the last year of their lives." (Tarkhnishvili, 1891, pp. 568–590.)

In the literature individual cases are described of persons who maintain active sex lives until the ages of 90–100. Some persons who married at these ages had children. Listed below are a few examples:

John Shell was born in 1788, married at the age of 19, and had 25 children. He married the second time at 125, and had a child from this marriage.

Nils Paulsen from Uppsala (Sweden) died in 1907 at the age of 160 years, leaving behind two sons, a 9-year-old boy and a 103-year-old man.

The English farmer Surrington lived to 160 years of age (1637–1797), and left children, the oldest of whom was 105 years, the youngest 9.

The Frenchman Longeville lived to 110 years and had 10 wives, marrying the last at the age of 99. His last wife bore him a son when he was 101 years old.

Thomas Parr, an English peasant, lived for 152 years and 9 months. He married for the first time at the age of 80 and had two children; he was married a second time at the age of 120 to a young widow, and from this marriage had a son who lived to the age of 123. On autopsy, the sex glands of Thomas Parr were found to be exceptionally well developed.

An unusual case was reported by the newspaper, *Pravda*, on September 19, 1964. In Ankara, the 95-year-old Turkish woman, Fatima Edirger, gave birth to twins, a boy and a girl; the father of the twins was 127 years old.

A. A. Bogomolets describes a visit by Henri Barbus in 1927 to the village of Laty near Sukhumi, where he met the peasant Shapkovski, who was then 140 years old. Barbus was surprised by Shapkovski's alertness, agility, strong voice, and clear eyes. Shapkovski's third wife was then 82 years old, and his youngest daughter was 25.

I. V. Bazilevich, a participant in two expeditions to Abkhazia, in his paper, "The Syndrome of Normal Senescence," (Bazilevich, 1940) cites data on the preservation of sexual attraction in the longliving at the ages of 90 and older. Many at this age have repeatedly married comparatively young women and had offspring from these marriages. For example, Datu Turkiya (109) was married for the third time at the age of 70 to an 18-year-old girl and had nine children from this marriage.

Mamsyr Kiut (117), after the death of his wife at the age of 92, no longer engaged in sex. His youngest daughter on the day of his death was 26.

Chubkar Shats (135) was married seven times, the last time at the age of 110. His youngest daughter was 13 years old.

Even in ancient times, reduced sexual activity was thought to be linked to the feebleness of old age. More than 2,000 years ago in China and India, the male sex glands of tigers and other animals were eaten as a remedy for senile impotency.

The experiments of Brown-Sekar using the infusion of a tincture from the seminal glands, those of Steinach involving the tying off of the seminiferous duct, and those of Voronov with implantation of testicles, are well known. Such interventions, however, were failures.

The reduction in the function of the sexual glands with the onset of old age has an effect upon the entire male organism, including work capacity and attitude. In light of the fact that the decline of testicular function occurs gradually, it is supposed that the male body can adapt to changes in the neurohormonal state. Therefore, such changes in men are not debilitating and are not accompanied by such upsetting symptoms as is sometimes the case in women. If in the past it was believed that the extinction of sexual function leads to the aging of the body, it is now well established that it is the aging of the body itself that is the cause of diminished sexual functioning.

The Tbilisi Gerontology Center, in collaboration with A. S. Agadzhanov, studied the sexual potency of the longliving of Georgia, along with marital status and numbers of children. The study was comprised of 222 males aged 100 years and older. The age distribution of the longliving in this study is presented in Table 11–1.

Table 11–1.

Age Distribution of Longliving Males of Soviet Georgia

Age (yrs.)	100–104	105–109	110–114	115–119	120–124	125	Total
No. of longliving	144	48	15	5	7	3	222

As early as 1925, I. I. Mechnikov wrote: "Sexual maturity, general physical maturity, and marital maturity (the age of marriage) are three important moments in human life which have one and the same goal—the satisfaction of the instinct for propagating the species (reproduction)." (Mechnikov, 1925, p. 49)

Of the 190 longliving males who indicated their marital status, only one was not married; the others had been married at different periods of their lives. The largest number of marriages took place at the age of 20–29 years (50.5%). Of the 189 longliving who were married, only four were childless; the others had numerous children.

As indicated in Table 11–2, the majority of the longliving had from four to six children (39.5%). Almost one-third of the longliving had from seven to nine children (30.3%), and only 25.4% had from one to three children, the others having more than 10 children (4.8%).

Table 11-2.

Number of Children of Longliving Males

No. of children	from 1 to 3	4 to 6	7 to 9	10 to 13
No. of longliving	47	73	56	9
	25.4%	39.5%	30.3%	4.8%

The birth of the last child as a function of the age of the father is interesting to note. As shown in Table 11–3, the largest number of children are born to the longliving at the age of 50–80 years (68.7%). Only two cases of the birth of children to longliving men aged 80–90 years are recorded.

Table 11-3.

Age of Longliving Males at Birth of Last Child

Age of longliving male at birth of last child (yrs.)	40–49	50–59	60–69	70–79	80–90
No. of longliving males	39	44	28	18	2
Percent of total	29.8%	33.6%	21.4%	13.7%	1.5%

Examples of the birth of offspring to longliving males who reached 100 years and older are provided by the following:

Z. V. Saralidze, born in 1861, from the village of Gelati of Lagodekh region; last child born when he was 86 years old.

M. O. Osmanov, born in 1848, from the villge of Munganlo of Dmanis region; had eight children, the last of whom was born when he was 80 years old.

Kh. Ts. Khurtskaya, born in 1838, from the village of Shamton of Zugdid region; had five children, the last of whom was born when he was 77 years old.

M. O. Azizbekov, born in 1860, from the village of Sadakhlo of Marneul region; had eight children, the last of whom was born when he was 76 years old.

Sexual potency of 180 longliving males were studied by the Tbilisi Gerontology Center. From Table 11–4, it is evident that even after the age of 80, 48.3% of the males retained their sexual potency. Moreover, in five of the longliving males, it was maintained even after the age of 100.

Table 11–4.

Sexual Potency of 180 Longliving Males

Age (yrs.)	60–69	70–79	80–89	90–99	100+
No. of sexually potent longliving males	168	97	67	25	5
Percent of total	93.3%	53.9%	37.2%	13.9%	2.8%

Below are listed longliving men who retained sexual potency.

I. A., Mskhiladze, born in 1860, from the village of Sabzar of the Adigen region; had three children, the last of whom was born in his 74th year. He retained sexual potency until the age of 100.

M. G. Tutberidze, born in 1836, from the village of Kviriti of the Telav region; had nine children, the last of whom was born when he was 61 years old. He retained sexual potency even after he had reached 100 years of age.

O. Kh. Piliya, born in 1839, from the Gudaut region; had five children, the last at the age of 62. Sexual potency was retained at the time of the examination.

A. A. Mikel, born in 1848, from the Marnelup region, village of Kachagan; had six children, the last born when he was 78. Sexual potency was retained at the time of the examination.

V. I. Chikurishvili, born in 1856, from the village of Napareuli, Telav region; had seven children, the last born when he was 57. He retained sexual potency up to the age of 100.

In 55% of the men, sexual potency was retained from ages of 80 to 100 years. Such a high percentage of retention of sexual potency indicated an active neuroendocrine system, and particularly, active hormonal function of the sex glands and the entire sexual system of the longliving men. This probably explains why sexual dysfunction appears much later in longliving men.

It is clear that provision for a regular sex life, along with a serious study of problems related to impotence and its treatment, are important areas for concern in the prolongation of life.

12

Prevention
and Treatment
of Premature
Aging

Concern for a long life should begin not when one has already passed 60, but at the time of birth, since childhood diseases leave their mark on one's entire life.

It is possible to prolong life and to extend the active socially productive period by combining sanitary-hygienic measures (social and personal hygiene) with biological intervention (hormones, vitamins, etc.). A high general standard of living, along with the health care and medical knowledge that usually accompany it, will allow everyone to maintain his or her health status by seeking early medical advice, and to retard the process of aging by rational control of his or her life.

The most important condition for longevity is a healthy nervous system. The cerebral cortex, which is the bearer of complex functions and subtle mechanisms, essentially reflects the sum total of changes in the internal and external environment. At the same time, it is a complex apparatus of harmonization and self-regulation of the bodily functions.

I. P. Pavlov wrote:

Our nervous system in the highest degree is self-regulating, self-supporting, self-restoring, self-correcting, and even self-improving. The most important, strongest and lasting impression of the study of the higher nervous activity by our method is the extreme plasticity of this activity, its tremendous possibilities: nothing remains stationary or inflexible and everything can always be achieved, changed for the better, once the appropriate conditions are realized. (1949, p. 454).

I. P. Pavlov believed that stress and exhaustion of the nervous system lead to diseases of various organs, as a result of which the metabolic processes are lowered, and a gradual withering of the cells and tissues occurs. Eventually a gradual slowing down and weakening of the entire body takes place. Therefore, it is important to guard against overstressing the nervous system.

Emotional experiences, especially negative emotions such as melancholy, sorrow, fear, envy, hate, and malice, greatly weaken normal body activity and the nervous system. The frequent experiencing of such emotions lead to the development of severe nervous disorders and the onset of premature aging. One must educate oneself in self-restraint, self-control; one must know how to suppress or to deal with negative emotions.

Meaningful relationships between people, emotional well-being, a pleasant disposition, enthusiasm, cheerfulness, self-control, and positive emotions all have a favorable influence upon human existence. Such positive emotions aid in the physiological equilibrium of the body and contribute to longevity. Finding enjoyment and satisfaction in work are also indications of good physical and mental health and a strong nervous system.

At the Ninth International Congress of Gerontologists in Kiev (1972), J. A. Hue stated that humankind should always be active, occupied with something. One does not have the right to lock oneself in a "mental ghetto," but should daily "open windows" to difficulties and joys. When the life-style is rigid, life is a heavy burden. When a life-style is selected voluntarily, considering circumstances, life is joy. The development of a series of recommendations for selecting a proper life-style—a life span perspective—should be the task of gerontologists of every nation.

Even Hippocrates—physician and philosopher who lived to the age of 104—recommended moderation, sensible gymnastics, fresh air, and walking for the prolongation of life. The famous Tadzhik scientist of the Middle Ages, Avicenna (Ibn Sina), placed a great value on the role of physical exercises for health and longevity. Participation in physical education and athletics has great preventive and therapeutic value.

Physical activity helped maintain the clarity of mind of L. N. Tolstoy, I. P. Pavlov, and I. Ye. Repin. They all walked and rode bicycles. Pavlov played skittles with his colleagues. Repin, while living in Kuokkala, when he picked up the mail at the station, distributed it to all his friends and acquaintances. Vladimir Ilich Lenin placed great value on physical exercise. In a letter to his sister, Mariya Ilinichna, he wrote: "Above all—do not forget your required daily gymnastics, force yourself to do several sets of tens (without yielding!) of all movements! This is very important" (n. d., p. 252).

In the Soviet Union, more than 3 million persons of middle and mature age participate in physical education and athletics. Special groups have been created for persons of mature and old age. However, physical activity cannot be separated from dietary habits. When assigning a set of physical exercises one should, at the same time, give recommendations regarding diet as well.

Brief daily morning and longer evening strolls and measured running are especially beneficial for the mature group. Such exercise promotes emotional equilibrium, alertness, and a bright mood. There is an International Association of Footracers of advanced age, with chapters in 27 countries. One veteran of this association is 89 years old and can run 5,000 meters in 39 minutes. The sportsmen of this association compete among one another in the marathon race, walkathons, and so on. The founder of the association, the German doctor Van Aachen, believes that prolonged walking, especially on forest paths with pauses, is the best remedy for obesity, circulatory disturbances, and rheumatism (Pointeau, 1972, pp. 24–25). Other forms of physical exercise are equally important, such as swimming, skating, skiing, hunting, fishing, and so forth.

In the modern age, people "live by nerve," and are prone to become overfatigued. At times, the nervous system becomes exhausted. Physical exercise—the alternation of walking, running, skiing, swimming, and other types of sports—leads to the activation of the entire muscular system and allows a full rest to the nervous system, thus alleviating overstress and overfatigue.

The healthful aspects of swimming are numerous. Regular participation in this sport develops and strengthens all the muscles, alleviates nervous fatigue, and restores strength. Healthy swimming at a moderate speed is a good preventive for heart disorders. This conclusion was reached by the participants in the symposium organized by the Medical Commission of the World Swimming Federation (FINA) in London. In health-club swimming pools, hundreds of elderly persons swim consistently. Physicians at these swimming clubs do not recall any instance in which swimming led to infarctions or other heart diseases. On the contrary, this type of sport has restored the health and working capacity of many elderly people or freed them from infarctions, neuroses, and psychoses. Regular physical exercise with a gradual load increase and observance of age-specific limitations, performed under medical surveillance, can overcome many syptoms of premature senescence in elderly people and strengthen the nervous system.

In order to build health, it is of great importance to use natural elements such as the sun, fresh air, and water. Studies have shown that atherosclerosis progresses rapidly in persons who do not avail themselves of the blessings of nature and lead "house-bound" lives. It is equally dangerous for people to avoid physical exercise, to "stuff themselves," and so on.

Nature is a natural guardian of health, an inexhaustible source of strength, health, and longevity. However, the gifts of nature should be used correctly for the purpose of strengthening the body, increasing the work capacity, and prolonging life. The observance of the rules of personal hygiene, sensible conditioning of the body by natural factors, such as sunbathing and mineral water baths, all aid in controlling diseases and the premature onset of aging. It is possible to recondition the body in all climatic zones and in all seasons.

The model of the Baku "health zone," managed by Prof. S. M. Gasanov, should be widely utilized (Gasanov, 1965). This modern therapeutic–physical exercise establishment was established in 1961. The zone covers the Revolution and Kirov parks, and the Primorye park, which extends 1.5 km. along the coast of the Caspian Sea, where the outpatient clinics and therapeutic facilities of the zone are located. The purpose of the "health zone" is to improve the health status of the total population, to provide restorative care, and to prolong human life. Wide use is made of the natural elements combined with an exercise program in the treatment of persons suffering from diseases of the cardiovascular, respiratory, and nervous systems.

The mature and old clients suffering from chronic diseases are not given drugs, but are treated through participation in hygienic gymnastics, therapeutic–physical exercises, and walking for prescribed distances and routes. Sea trips on launches, air and sun baths, and time spent at the seashore are all prescribed and monitored by the physician.

Additional treatment and physical conditioning is provided through phytotherapy (treatment with the odors of different flowers), as well as hydrotherapy, physiotherapy, and music therapy.

The health measures employed in industry, including sanitation and safety precautions, have significantly reduced the total morbidity of workers, along with temporary loss of work capacity, occupational diseases, and injury rate. Despite the constant improvements in working conditions, however, occupational pollution is still present in a number of industries: noise, vibration, dust, and gases all have a deleterious effect upon the health of the workers, resulting in a shortened life span. Industries employing older workers need to pay particular heed to the pollution level and to develop appropriate working conditions. Occupations that involve a high degree of nervous tension need to develop scheduling in which work and rest periods are balanced. When older workers are involved, such scheduling should include prolonged rest breaks, allowing for bodily functions to be restored.

ALCOHOLISM

Two hundred years ago, M. V. Lomonosov, in a letter to Count Shuvalov, outlined quite clearly the consequences of drunkenness. In Russia at the time of Peter the First, drunkards were imprisoned for their transgressions, and a medal weighing 6 kg, 800 gm with the inscription, "For Drunkenness," was hung about the necks of those who continued to drink, until the end of their term of incarceration.

In the Soviet Union today, alcoholism is still a problem among certain societal groups. Alcoholism undermines health and accelerates the aging process, as it disturbs the normal functions of the nervous system, inflicting irreparable damage. Abuse of alcohol significantly decreases the vital activities of the body, making it susceptible to diseases, lowering the resistance, and reducing the working capacity. The systematic ingestion of alcohol also affects the heart muscle, leading to sclerotic changes and significantly weakening its functional capacity. The excessive use of alcohol leads to paralysis of the centers of attention and self-control.

SMOKING

Smoking exerts a harmful effect on all organs and tissues of the body. Among smokers, besides lung cancer and myocardial infarction, there are also found cancer of the larynx, peptic and duodenal ulcers, cancer of the urinary bladder, and severe liver lesions.

Nicotine damages the nervous system, above all causing its overstressing with subsequent exhaustion. Abuse of smoking causes a chronic overexcitation of the nervous system, resulting in the development of neurasthenia, a weakening of the memory, disturbances in the senses of smell and taste, and a severe weakening of the senses of vision and hearing.

Besides the toxic effects of the nicotine contained in tobacco on the organs of circulation, respiration, and on the nervous system, among heavy smokers of long duration have been found cases of chronic intoxication, leading to premature aging, emaciation, typical changes in the lines of the face, and a shortening of the average life expectancy.

The average life expectancy of smokers is 25% lower than that of nonsmokers. Kyler Hammond (United States) calculated that the chances of living to 65 and longer are 78% for nonsmoking men at the age of 25, and only 54% for men of the same age smoking 40 or more cigarettes per day. (Hammond and Horn, 1956, p. 69)

Smoking should be stopped immediately without tapering down. This may appear to be difficult, but it is possible to accomplish. Giving up smoking will restore health, increase energy and work capacity, and prolong life.

PERSONAL HYGIENE

One should be concerned about the cleanliness of the skin, bathing no less frequently than once a week. Care of the body should begin with the skin. According to I. P. Pavlov, the skin is the oldest and most reliable intermediary between the organism and the environment.

BREATHING AND FRESH AIR

In workplaces proper ventilation should be maintained. If the air of the area becomes contaminated by tobacco smoke, it may be especially harmful for nonsmokers, who have not developed a resistance to nicotine. Consequently, it is very important to ventilate the establishment on a regular basis.

One should breathe deeply so that the exhaled air is not retained in the lungs, allowing the blood to be enriched with oxygen.

SLEEP

In the daily schedule, a proper amount of time should be devoted to sleep—the primary form of rest. I. P. Pavlov calls sleep the "saviour of our nervous system." It is calculated that human beings spend about 23 years of their lives sleeping—that is, almost one-third.

The outstanding Georgian physiologist, I. R. Tarkhnishvili, demonstrated through his experiments that insomnia is more dangerous than starvation. An animal that had not received food for 25 days remained alive, while a dog that was not allowed to sleep died within 5 days.

Without a normal full night's sleep, one cannot be healthy or expect to prolong one's life. This is especially true in the contemporary era, a period of rapid technological and cultural change, fraught with psychological stress and emotional strain, amidst an avalanche of new and varied information. These conditions, coupled with other factors that impinge on the body, not only shorten the period of nightly rest, but bring about restlessness and intermittent sleep. Systematic sleep deprivation and insomnia lead to severe nervous disorders and a drop in working capacity.

Sleep provides the organism with a total rest, restoring the working capacity as well as the normal tonus and resistance of the nervous system.

One should go to bed and get up at a certain specific time, stopping intellectual work 1.5 to 2 hours before sleep, and not eating just before sleep. After middle-age, among the mature, sleep should not last longer than 9–10 hours, and in old age and in the longliving, it should consist of night sleep and a brief afternoon nap.

In order to improve or induce sleep, strolling in the evenings is recommended, no matter what the weather. One should sleep with an open window. After awakening, one should feel fully refreshed and capable of work. In cases of sleep disorders, one should consult a physician, who will ascertain the cause and prescribe the appropriate treatment.

SEXUAL ACTIVITY

Sexual hygiene has great significance for health and longevity.

The Venetian nobleman, L. Kornaro, in his treatise, *Experience on the benefit of a sober life* (1558) wrote of the deleterious effect of sexual profligacy on the health and duration of life. He emphasized the fact that drunkenness and "excessive lovemaking" undermine the health, causing premature aging. Kornaro, like the majority of youthful Italian nobility of that time, had led the life of a libertine and indulged heavily in food and alcoholic beverages. Drastically changing his life-style, Kornaro lived to the age of 98, preserving good health and intellect.

Ch. Hufeland, in the book, *The art of prolonging human life: macrobiotics* (1796), called attention to the need for a normalized sexual life. He believed that people who lived to advanced old age never abused their sexual capacities, but engaged in moderate sexual activity. These assertions of Ch. Hufeland have not lost their importance with time.

PHARMACOLOGY AND AGING

In recent years, drugs have been developed that counteract the onset of premature aging and improve the general tonus of the entire organism. Efforts have been directed toward the production of drugs that will alleviate memory loss and control depressive states. Drugs have been synthesized that actively normalize the blood pressure and dissolve thrombi at the point where irreversible tissue lesions arise.

However, the elderly organism reacts differently to the drugs ingested; therefore, the doses of such drugs should be considerably reduced when they are prescribed. Among the drugs that reduce the manifestation of the various pathological processes in the elderly and improve their general condition is novocaine. The effect of novocaine or procaine is equivalent to that of vitamins. It contains hydrochloride of the diethylaminoethyl ether of para-aminobenzoic acid. However, the effect of novocaine on the elderly organism is produced not only by the action of this acid but principally by its neurotrophic effect.

A. Aslan believes that novocaine acts on the body through the nervous system via neuroendocrine correlations and through the vascular system and metabolic processes. In the Soviet Union good results have been obtained in the prevention of premature aging and in treating certain diseases of mature and older persons with the Romanian preparation Gerovital. This drug represents a vitaminized 2% procaine solution, stabilized and tamponated by the method of A. Aslan. Besides using Gerovital for the prevention of premature aging, it is also used in the treatment of some senile disorders. (Parkhon, 1959, p. 423)

Studies conducted on patients aged 60 years and older have led to the conclusion that Gerovital is effective in the treatment of the initial forms of atherosclerosis, when functional shifts predominate over organic ones. As a result of the treatment, the activity of the cardiovascular system of the patients improved; the unpleasant feelings in the region of the heart vanished, while the cholesterol level, the lecithin-cholesterol index, and the prothrombin index normalized (Pitskhelauri & Saakadze, 1968).

Gerovital treatment is more effective when combined with vitamins, hormones, and the like. In mature and old age, and in the longliving, the coefficient of utilization of the vitamins from food products declines; this significantly increases their requirement in order to offset the decline in energy potential of the aging cell.

Vitamins and vitamin complexes properly administered have an obvious role in the general stimulation of the elderly organism. These substances increase the tonus of the physiological processes and the reactivity of the organism. The specific effect of vitamins consists in the fact that, as they are a part of the composition of more than 100 enzymes, they promote activation of the metabolic processes, while exercising a substantial effect on the protein, lipid, carbohydrate, and water-mineral metabolism. Besides this, vitamins participate in the formation of the macroergic compounds, mediators, hormones, antibodies—thereby stimulating the processes of regeneration and general reactivity of the body.

In the aging organism, a deficiency of many vitamins is detected, but primarily that of ascorbic acid and a number of vitamins of the B group. Vitamins should be prescribed predominantly for oral ingestion, since the digestive system, when in satisfactory condition, has the protective property of shielding against possible vitamin over-doses (Chebotarev, 1966).

In recent years, the Institute of Gerontology of the USSR Academy of Medical Sciences has been conducting studies of the effect not only of individual vitamins, but also of vitamin complexes on the aging organism. Among the effective vitamin complexes proposed by the Institute, one should mention "Dekamevit" (Virgerin) and "Undevit." However, all of these agents should be used by prescription and under medical control, with the observance of all the general rules of health.

MEDICAL CARE

Untended or undiagnosed diseases are the cause of unfortunate losses of valuable members of the work force. The advice of physicians should be sought upon the first symptoms and signs of disabilities. This is especially true with regard to the mature and old-aged persons.

Particular attention should be devoted to the prevention of diseases of the heart and vessels. Cardiovascular diseases are closely related to disturbances in work and rest and life-style, to harmful habits, and to disruptions of dietary laws. In this connection, proper precautions for the prevention of heart and vessel diseases have been advanced by the leading American cardiologist Paul White, the first winner of the International Gold Stethoscope prize:

1. Do not use an automobile in the city; walk or ride a bicycle.
2. Do not smoke.
3. Keep your weight the same as it was at the age of 22 (It is well known, for example, that overweight persons experience coronary insufficiency twice as often).
4. The development in as early as the elementary grades of an optimistic and outgoing attitude. Even A. A. Bogomolets said: "One of the factors of longevity is courtesy and pleasant relationships with people."

Such observations clearly demonstrate that each of us can slow down the aging process.

RETIREMENT

Old persons who are capable of work and who have accumulated rich experiences in the course of several decades, along with practical wisdom and deep moral strength, are valuable capital for society. The wisdom of the elderly was highly valued in ancient times. Solon, the legendary legislator of the Greek people, believed that the old man is made wise by his life's experience, knows people well with their weaknesses and transgressions, and can be unimpassioned and just in judgment. Solon the Wise entrusted the "last court of appeal," above which there were only the gods, not to the young, not to the middle-aged, and not to the mature citizens of Athens, but to the very old men. The court procedure consisted in the old men's climbing the hill of Ares and constituting the bench called the Areopagus where they pronounced their sentences on criminals, not only according to the letter of the law, but also according to "moral conviction."

The increase in the average life expectancy in the Soviet Union, along with the activity level of persons of mature and very old age, are indications that many persons who are of retirement age and even older, continue to be productive. Such continued activity is especially true of persons within the more intellectually demanding professions. In light of these facts, we need to reconsider the notion of age limits with respect to real capacities of persons to perform physical and intellectual work.

At the same time, the "third age" requires not only medical but also social assistance, and above all the development of a positive attitude toward the elderly on the part of family members and social organizations.

The process of adaptation for elderly people who have retired is a serious problem. The sudden cessation of work that formed much of the life of the retired person, in many cases, is difficult to endure. The stress of adapting to new living conditions, the breaking of the accustomed routine, sometimes leads to a mental breakdown, isolation, or loneliness. Therefore, the problem of the social welfare agencies, public organizations, the family, and friends is to provide support to retired persons during the adaptation process.

B. D. Petrov, emphasizing the urgency of the problem of adaptation of elderly people with regard to retirement, believes that this problem requires particular attention and includes several components: the psychological, physiological, and sociological. An attentive and careful study of the nature of adaptation to new living conditions by retirees of various occupations and different social positions is necessary in order to provide them with suitable work opportunities whenever possible. (Petrov, 1972, p. 227)

To maintain the working capacity of mature and old persons, to promote the reasonable use of these capabilities, and to encourage their ability to utilize their life's experience toward the goal of prolonging life—constitute an important mission for society.

References

Alikishiev, R. Sh. Longevity in Dagestan, in *Problems of longevity*. Academy of Sciences: Moscow, 1962.

Arnold of Villanova. *Regimen sanitatis salernitanum* (tr. from Latin with remarks by Yu. F. Shults). Moscow, 1970.

Atlas of Georgia. Tibilisi, 1965.

Bagrationi, I. *Collected medical works*. Manuscript No. 136, Manuscript Dept. of the Leningrad Institute for Oriental Studies.

Bazilevich, I. V. The normal aging symdrome, in *Aging: Proceedings of the conference on the genesis of aging and the prevention of premature aging, Kiev, 17–19 December, 1938*. USSR Academy of Sciences: Kiev, 1940.

Bebel, A. *Future society*. 1959.

Bednyy, M. S. *Demographic processes and predictions of the health of the population*. Moscow, 1972.

Binet, L., & Bourlier, F. (Eds.). *Principles of gerontology*. Medical Literature: Moscow, 1960.

Bogatyrev, I. D. Medical and social aspects in the care of the elderly. *Proceedings of the 9th international congress on gerontology*, Chebotarev, D. F., ed. Kiev: 1972, v. 3.

Bourlier, F. *Aging and senescence: principles of hygiene and therapy* (tr. from French). Moscow, 1962.

Celsus, A. C. *On medicine* (vols.). Moscow, 1959.

Chebotarev, D. F., Frolkis, V. V., & Mankovski, N. B. Aging and Physiological systems of the organism. In *Papers of the 2nd All-Union Conference of Gerontologists and Geriatricians*, December 9–11, 1969.

Chernyshevskiy, N. G. *Chto delat?*

Davydovsky, I. V. *Gerontology*. Moscow, 1966.

Dublin, L., & Lotka, A. New York: 1936.

The formula for the elixir of long life and its properties. M. E. Saltikov-Schedrin Public Library, Code No. 18.207.1.294.

Frenkel, Z. G. *Prolonging life and active old age.* Moscow, 1949.

Gasanov, S. M. *Central Baku health zone.* Baku, 1965.

Geratsi, M. *Utesheniye pri likhoradkakh (Treatment of fever).* Yerevan, 1968.

Grombakh, S. M. *Russian medical literature of the XVIII century.* Moscow, 1953, p. 278.

Hammond, K. E. and Horn, D. D., the relationship between smoking habits and death, *The journal of health and welfare*, no. 1, 1956.

Hippocrates. *On diet.* In *Works II*, Book 1, para. 33.

Hufeland, Ch. *The art of prolonging human life: macrobiotics.* (1796)

Jalavista, E. An inheritance of longevity according to Finnish and Swedish geneaologies. *Annal of Finnish Medical Experiments*, 1951, **40**, 263-274.

Kadyan, A. A. Population of St. Petersburg municipal almshouses. In *Materials for the study of senescence according to research conducted under the leadership of S. P. Botkin in 1889.* St. Petersburg, 1890.

Kananeli. *Ustsoro Karabadini.* Tbilisi, 1940, p. 339.

Kopili, K. *Tsigni saakimoi.* Tbilisi, 1936, p. 40.

Kurkin, P. I. Problems of sanitary statistics. In A. M. Merkov (Ed.), *Selected works.* Moscow, 1961.

Laroche, K., & Bourlier, F.

Lenin, V. I. *Works*, Vol 37.

Marshak, M. S. *Sovetskoye zakonodatistvo (Soviet legislation).* 1959, No. 12, p. 25.

Mechnikov, I. I. *Forty year search for a rational world view.* State Printing Office: Moscow, 1925

Niel, D., & Shell, V. *Human heredity*, BME, Moscow, 1961.

Nagorny, A. V., Nikitin, V. N., & Bulankin, I. N. *Problems of aging and longevity.* V. N. Nikitin, ed. Moscow, 1963.

Novoselskiy, S.

Panaskerteli-Tsitsishvili, Z. *Samkurnalo tsigni*, Parts I & II (M. Shengeliya, Ed.). Tbilisi, 1950, 1959.

Parkhon, K. I. *Biology of Aging.* Foreign Language Editions: Bucharest, 1959.

Pavlov, I. P. *Conditioned reflexes*, BTE, Vol. 30.

Pavlov, I. P. *Full collected works*, Vols. 3 (1st ed.). 1949.

Pavlov, I. P. *Pavlovian environments*, Vol. 1. AN USSR, 1949.

Pavlov, I. P. *Selected works.* 1951.

Pearl, R. Experiments in longevity. *Quarterly Review of Biology*, 1938, 3, 391–401.

Petrov, B. D. Adaptation to new living conditions in retirement, in *Proceedings of the 9th international congress on gerontology*, Chebotarev, D. F., ed. Kiev, 1972.

Petrovskiy, B. Statement at 31st session of General Convention of USSR Academy of Medical Sciences. *Vestnik Akademii Meditsinskikh Nauk*, 1971, **12**, 67.

Pineau, G. *Philosophy of longevity.* St. Petersburg, 1901.

Pisarev, D. I. School and life. 1865.

Pitskhelauri, G. Z. *The contribution of I. R. Tarkhnishvili to the problem of longevity and senescence.* Tbilisi, 1968.

Pitskhelauri, G. Z. Patho-anatomical section by W. Harvey of the body of Thomas Parr. *Arkhiv patologii (Pathological Archives)*, 1963, No. 3.

Pitskhelauri, G. Z., & Dzhorbenadze, D. A. Scholars of medieval Georgia on senescence and longevity. *Zdravoo Khraneniye (International Journal)*, Bucharest, 1969, p. 4.

Pitskhelauri, G. Z., & Saakadze, V. I. Gerovital in the treatment of atherosclerosis in persons of mature and old age. *Controlling Premature Aging*, Kiev, 1968.

Pointeau, R. *Zdorov ye mira (World Health)*, July 1972, pp. 24–25.

Rolland, R. *Collected works*, Vol. 14.

Rosset, E. *The process of aging of the population: demographic study.* (tr. from Polish). Moscow, 1968.

Rubakin, A. N. *In praise of old age.* Moscow, 1966.

Sachuk, N. N. (Ed.). *Proceedings of the 9th International Congress of Gerontology*, Vol. 2. July 2–7, 1972, Kiev.

Senescence. *Papers of the Conference on the Problem of the Onset of Senescence and the Prevention of Premature Aging of the Organism*, December 17–19, 1938. Kiev, 1940.

Shapiro, I. B., Pitskhelauri, G. Z., & Gagua, O. Ye. *The oldest people of Tbilisi*. Tbilisi, 1956.

Spasokukotskiy, U. A. *Prevention of premature aging.* Kiev, 1968.

Tarkhnishvili, I. R. Doctors of centenarian age of all times and peoples. *Vestnik i biblioteka samoobrazovaniya (Herald and library self-education). Khronika (Chronicle)*, 1903.

Tarkhnishvili, I. R. Longevity in animals, plants and humans. *European Herald*, St. Petersburg, 1891, Index V–XI, N. 5, 136–163.

United Nations. *Demographic reference book*, 1970.

Urlanis, B. Ts. *Birth rate and human life expectancy in the USSR.* Moscow, 1963.

World Health Organization. *Minutes of Seminar*, Copenhagen, 1963.

World population reference manual. Moscow, 1965.

Yules, M. and Khello, I., *Diagnosis and pathophysiological symptoms of neuroendocrinological illnesses*.

Zhordaniya, I. F. (Ed.), *Infertile marriage*, Vol. 1. Tbilisi, 1960.

BIBLIOGRAPHY

Atlas of Georgia. Tbilsi, 1964. Soviet Georgia Academy of Science.

Bagrationi, I. *Collected medical works*. Manuscript No. 136, Manuscript Dept. of the Leningrad Institute for Oriental Studies.

Bebel, A. *Future society*. 1959.

Bednyy, M. S. *Demographic processes and predictions of the health of the population*. Moscow, 1972.

Benet, S. *Abkhasians: the long living people of the Caucasus*. New York: Holt, Rinehart & Winston, 1974.

Benet, S. *How to live to be 100*. New York: Dial Press, 1976.

Berdishev, G. D. *Ecological-hygienic factors of aging and longevity*. Leningrad, 1968.

Binet, L., & Bourlier, F. (Eds.). *Principles of gerontology*. Medical Literature/Moscow, 1960.

Binstock, R. (Ed.). *Proceedings of the 9th International Congress on Gerontology*, Chebotarev, D. F., ed. Vol. 1, Kiev, 1972, p. 222.

Bourlier, F. *Aging and senescence: principles of hygiene and therapy* (tr. from French). Moscow, 1962.

Celsus, A. C. *On medicine* (8 vols.). Moscow, 1959.

Chebotarev, D. F., Vitamins in the prevention and treatment of atherosclerosis, in *Vitamins in the prevention and treatment of premature aging*. Health: Kiev, 1966, p. 9.

Chebotarev, D. F. *Prevention of premature aging*. Kiev, 1960, p. 660.

Chebotarev, D. F. *Longevity*. Moscow, 1970, p. 18.

Chebotarev, D. F. "The socio-hygienic aspects of gerontology," *Soviet Health Care*, 1972, **7**, 3–9.

Chebotarev, D. F. *Guide to gerontology*. Moscow, 1978.

Chebotarev, D. F., Frolkis, V. V., & Mankovski, N. B. Aging and physiological systems of the organism. In *Papers of the 2nd All-Union Conference of Gerontologists and Geriatricians*. December 9–11, 1969.

Chebotarev, D. F. Frolkis, V. V., & Mankovski, N. B. *Foundations of gerontology*. Moscow, 1969.

Comfort, A. *Biology of aging*. Moscow, 1967, p. 398.

Davidenkov, S., & Efroimson, V. *Human heredity*, BME, Vol. XIX. Soviet Encyclopedia: Moscow, 1961, p. 1009.

Davydovsky, I. V. *Gerontology.* Moscow, 1966.

Dublin, L., & Lotka, A. New York: 1936.

Dzhavakhishvili, A. N. *Population density and settlement distribution according to elevation in the Georgian Caucasus,* Publication of the Geographical Society of Soviet Georgia: Tbilisi, 1963, V. vii, p. 55.

Dzorbenadze, D. A. (Ed.). *Proceedings of the 9th International Congress of Gerontology,* Vol. 3, Kiev, 1972, p. 203.

Engels, F. *Origin of the family.* 1950, p. 133.

The formula for the elixir of long life and its properties. M. E. Saltikov-Schedrin Public Library, Code No. 18.207.1.294.

Frenkel, Z. G. *Prolonging life and active old age.* Moscow, 1949.

Gasanov, S. M. *Central Baku health zone.* Baku, 1965.

Gensac, G. *We will live to be 100.* Editions Mendiales. Paris: 1960.

Jalavista, E. An inheritance of longevity according to Finnish and Swedish geneaologies. *Annal of Finnish Medical Experiments,* 1951, **40,** 263–274.

Kadyan, A. A. Population of St. Petersburg municipal almshouses. In *Materials for the study of senescence according to research conducted under the leadership of S. P. Botkin in 1889.* St. Petersburg, 1890.

Kananeli. *Ustsoro karabadini.* Tbilisi, 1940.

Kipshidze, N. N., & Chapidze, G. E. *Contemporary problems in gerontology and geriatrics.* Tbilisi, 1977, pp. 363–365

Kopili, K. *Tsigni saakimoi.* Tbilisi, 1936.

Kornaro, L. *Experience on the benefit of a sober life.* 1558.

Kosinskaya, N. C., and Makkaveiski, P. A. Aging: Proceedings of the 3rd Conference on the Causes and Prevention of Premature Aging, Kiev, 1940.

Krikov, F. G. "Hygienic problems in the amelioration of the natural human environment," *Academy of Medical Science News,* 1971, 12, 67.

Kurkin, P. I. Problems of sanitary statistics. In A. M. Merkov (Ed.) *Selected works.* Moscow, 1961.

Leaf, A. "Every day is a gift when you are over 100," *National Geographic,* January 1973, **143** (no. 1), 93–119.

Leaf, A. *Youth in old age.* New York: McGraw-Hill, 1975.

Lenin, V. I. *Collected works.* (4th ed.) Political Literature: Leningrad, 1952, p. 229.

Lenin, V. I. *Works,* Political Literature: Leningrad. Vol. 37. 252.

Lesnoff-Caravaglia, G. *Health care of the elderly.* New York: Human Sciences Press, 1980.

Marshak, M. S. *Sovetskoye Zakonodatlstvo (Soviet legislation).* 1959, No. 12, p. 25.

McKain, Walter C. "Are They Really That Old? Some Observations Concerning Extreme Old Age in the Soviet Union," *The Gerontologist*, Vol. 7, No. 1, 1967, 70–73.

—————. "Fertility and Longevity," *Omega*, Vol. 7(4), 1976–77, 361–365.

—————. "The Zone of Health," *The Gerontologist*, Vol. 9, No. 1, Spring, 1969, 47–54.

Mikhtar, G. *Treatment of fevers*. Yerevan, 1968. p. 121.

Morisita, I. K. *Secrets of the incredible longliving people of Georgia*. Tokyo, 1980.

Myllymaki, P. *Sata vuotiaat*. Helsinki: 1967.

Nagorny, A. V., Nikitin, V. N., & Bulankin, I. N. *Problems of aging and longevity*. Medical Literature Series, V. N. Nikitin, ed. Moscow, 1963.

Panaskerteli-Tsitsishvili, Z. *Karabadini medical manual*. Tbilisi, 1978.

Parkhon, K. I. *Biology of aging*. Bucharest, 1960.

Pavlov, I. P. *Conditioned reflexes*, BTE, Vol. 3.

Pavlov, I. P. *Full collected works* Vol. 3. Academy of Sciences, USSR. (1st ed.). 1949.

Pavlov, I. P. *Pavlovian environments*, Vol. 1. Academy of Sciences, USSR, 1949.

Pavlov, I. P. *Selected works*. 1951.

Pearl, R. Experiments in longevity. *Quarterly Review of Biology*, 1938, 3, 391–401.

Petrov, B. D. Adaptation to new living conditions in retirement, in *Proceedings of the 9th International Congress on Gerontology*, vol. II, D. F. Chebotarev, ed. Kiev, 1972, p. 227.

Pineau, G. *Philosophy of longevity*. St. Petersburg, 1901.

Pitskhelauri, G. Z. Patho-anatomical section by W. Harvey of the body of Thomas Parr. *Arkhiv patologii (Pathological Archives)*, 1963, No. 3.

—————. *The contribution of I. R. Tarkhnishvili to the problem of longevity and senescence*. Tbilisi, 1968.

—————. *Hygiene and Health*, 1968, **7,**

—————. Some socio-demographic changes in the population of the long-living of Soviet Georgia. *Gerontology and Geriatrics*, Kiev, 1973.

—————. *The longliving of Soviet Georgia*. Tbilisi, 1976.

—————. *Materials from the First Assembly of Georgian Hygiene and Health Officers*. Tbilisi, 1976, pp. 515–517.

Pitskhelauri, G. Z. *Contemporary problems in gerontology and geriatrics*. Tbilisi, 1977.

—————. *Life-styles and health*. Moscow, 1977.

—————. *The longliving of Soviet Georgia*. Tbilisi, 1978.

Pitskhelauri, G. Z., Dueli, L., Dzorbenadze, D. A., Agadzhanov, A. S., & Eyderman, M. M. *Collected works of I. F. Zhordaniya on the physiology and pathology of women.* Tbilisi, 1969.

Pitskhelauri, G. Z., Dueli, L., & Stepanov, P. *Problems of gerontology and geriatrics in orthopedics and traumatology.* Kiev, 1966.

Pitskhelauri, G. Z., & Dzhorbenadze, D. A. *Scholars of medieval Georgia on senescence and longevity. Zdravoo Khraneniye (International Journal),* Bucharest, 1969, 9.

Pitskhelauri, G. Z., & Pivovarova, I. P. *Gerohygiene in the 9th International Congress on Gerontology,* Vol. 1. Soviet Ministry of Health, 1974.

Pitskhelauri, G. Z., & Saakadze, V. I. Gerovital in the treatment of athrosclerosis in persons of mature and old age. *Controlling Premature Aging.* Kiev, 1968. p. 81.

Proceedings of the VOZ Seminar, Chebotarev, D. F. ed. Copenhagen, 1963.

Pointeau, R. *Zclorov ye mira (World Health),* "Sports for all Ages" July 1972, pp. 24–25.

Rolland, R. *Collected works,* Vol. 14. Moscow: Soviet Writers, 1939.

Rosset, E. *The process of aging of the population: demographic study* (tr. from Polish). Moscow, 1968.

Rubakin, A. N. *In praise of old age.* Moscow, 1966.

Sachuk, N. N. Socio-demographic characteristics of the elderly population of the USSR, in *Lifestyles of the elderly.* Kiev, 1966, pp. 8–19.

Sachuk, N. N. (Ed.). *Proceedings of the 9th International Congress of Gerontology,* Vol. 2. Chebotarev, D. F., ed. July 2–7, 1972, Kiev.

Serenko, A. F., Ermakov, V. V., & Petrakov, V. D. *Foundations for the organization of polyclinic assistance for a population.* Moscow, 1976.

Shapiro, I. B., Pitskhelauri, G. Z., & Gagua, O. Ye. *The oldest people of Tbilisi.* Tbilisi, 1956.

Shults, Yu. F. *Health code of Salerno* (Tr. with commentary from the Latin). Moscow, 1970.

Spasokukotskiy, U. A. *Prevention of premature aging.* Kiev, 1968.

Spasokukochkii, U. A., Barchenko, L. I., and Gennis, E. D., *Longevity and physiological aging.* USSR State Medical Publications: Kiev, 1963, pp. 33–34.

Strehler, B. *Time, cells and aging.* Moscow, 1964.

Tarkhnishvili, I. R. Doctors of centenarian age of all times and peoples. *Vestnik i biblioteka samoobrazovaniya (Herald and Library Self-Education). Khronika (Chronicle),* 1903.

Tarkhnishvili, I. R. Longevity in animals, plants and humans. *In European Herald.* Thought: St. Petersburg, 1891, No. 5, pp. 136–163.

United Nations. *Demographic reference book*, 1970.

United Nations Department of Population Studies. *Population growth estimates according to age, socio-economic status, region and nation*, 1965–1985.

Urlanis, B. Ts. *Birth rate and human life expectancy in the USSR*. Moscow, 1963.

Vilenchik, M. M. *Molecular mechanisms of aging*. Moscow, 1970.

Vinogradov, N. A., & Revutskaya, Z. G. *Main problems of Soviet gerontology*. Kiev, 1972, pp. 263–276.

Voronov, S. A. *Life extension*. Moscow, 1933.

World population reference manual. Moscow, 1965.

Yengalychev, P. *On prolonging human life*. Smirdinna Printers: St. Petersburg, 1825. 1801.

Zhordaniya, I. F. (Ed.). *Infertile marriage*, Vol. 1. Tbilisi, 1960.

Zhordaniya, I. F. *Collected works (NII) physiology and pathology*. Tbilisi, 1969.

Index